Engaging and Communicating
with People Who Have Dementia

Engaging and Communicating with People Who Have Dementia

Finding and Using Their Strengths

by

Eileen Eisner, M.ED., CCC-SLP

with invited contributions by

Michelle S. Bourgeois, M.S., PH.D., CCC-SLP
Joan L. Green, M.A., CCC-SLP

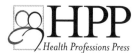

Baltimore • London • Sydney

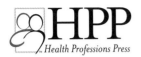
HPP
Health Professions Press

Health Professions Press, Inc.
Post Office Box 10624
Baltimore, Maryland 21285-0624

www.healthpropress.com

Interior and cover designs by Mindy Dunn.
Typeset by Barton Matheson Willse & Worthington, Baltimore, Maryland.
Manufactured in the United States of America by Versa Press, East Peoria, Illinois.

This book is a revised edition of the previously titled *Can Do Activities for Adults with Alzheimer's Disease: Strength-Based Communication and Programming* (Eisner, 2001).

Library of Congress Cataloging-in-Publication Data

Eisner, Eileen, author.
   Engaging and communicating with people who have dementia : finding and using their strengths / by Eileen Eisner.
      p. ; cm.
   Based on: Can do activities for adults with Alzheimer's disease : strength-based communication and programming / Eileen Eisner. Pro-Ed. c2001.
   Includes bibliographical references and index.
   ISBN 978-1-938870-03-3
   I. Eisner, Eileen. Can do activities for adults with Alzheimer's disease. Based on (work): II. Title.
   [DNLM: 1. Alzheimer Disease. 2. Communication. 3. Needs Assessment. WT 155]
   RC524
   616.8'31—dc23
                                                                                    2013026933

British Library Cataloguing in Publication data are available from the British Library.

When words and memories fade, love remains.

This book is dedicated in memory of my mother,
Bert Goldstein, in honor of my father, Herbert Goldstein,
and with love and appreciation to my husband, Averell Eisner.

———————————

*The advantage of a bad memory is that, several times over,
one enjoys the same good things for the first time.*
—Friedrich Nietzsche

Contents

Informal Geriatric Strength-Based Inventory

Caregiver Questionnaire and Checklist

Personal Preferences Inventory

Strength-Based Summary Sheet

SIMPLE (Simplified Inventory of Multiple Potential and Leisure Engagement)

Dementia Care Staff Guide

Memory Loss Caregiver Guide

About the Author
and Contributors

Eileen Eisner, M.Ed., CCC-SLP, is a speech-language pathologist with more than 30 years of experience. She specializes in communication disorders related to Alzheimer's disease, as well as language-learning disorders in school-age children. Eisner is the author of *Merging Language Intervention with Classroom Practices: A Guide for the Speech-Language Pathologist* (1998), and *Can Do Activities for Adults with Alzheimer's Disease: Strength-Based Communication and Programming* (2001). She served as the Director of Speech and Language Services of Westfield, NJ. Eisner has presented papers at both the state and national meetings of the American Speech-Language-Hearing Association as well as the Alzheimer's Association. A seasoned consultant, Eisner has written professional articles on practical intervention strategies for adults who have neurodegenerative dementias and also provides staff training sessions on the strategies.

Michelle S. Bourgeois, M.S., Ph.D., CCC-SLP, is Professor in the Department of Speech and Hearing Science at The Ohio State University. Her teaching interests include adult language disorders, including with respect to dementia and traumatic brain injury. A clinical researcher, Dr. Bourgeois has investigated interventions for spousal and nursing home caregivers designed to improve the quality and quantity of communicative interactions, the evaluation of memory aids for persons with dementia and traumatic brain injury, and the development of training programs for institutional caregivers. Dr. Bourgeois has published numerous research articles, training manuals and CDs, and books, including *Memory and Communication Aids for People with Dementia* (Health Professions Press, 2013).

Joan L. Green, M.A., CCC-SLP, is a licensed and certified speech-language pathologist with many years of experience helping individuals of all ages who have communication, cognitive, literacy, and learning challenges to maximize progress and enhance their overall quality of life. The founder of Innovative

Speech Therapy, Green has developed a new and effective approach to therapy using technology and other unique resources to empower individuals, families, and professionals with state-of-the-art treatment. She coaches professionals, students, clients, and caregivers at the local, state, and national levels on integrating computers and technology into SLP treatment. She is the author of *The Ultimate Guide to Assistive Technology in Special Education: Resources for Education, Intervention, and Rehabilitation* (2011), and *Technology for Communication and Cognitive Treatment: The Clinician's Guide* (2007). Green also offers an informative free e-newsletter to more than 7,000 professionals and families that highlights strategies using technology to help maximize progress toward goals.

Acknowledgments

I wish to acknowledge the significant contribution made to this book by Susan Harris, CEO of the Oscar and Ella Wilf Campus for Senior Living in Somerset, New Jersey. Susan graciously shared her expertise and time. I also want to acknowledge Char Christensen, activities director for First Community Village in Columbus, Ohio; Dakim, Inc., of Santa Monica, California; and Michelle S. Bourgeois, Ph.D., of The Ohio State University Speech & Hearing Clinic, for their efforts in providing many of the chapter photographs.

Preface

As an intuitive speech-language pathologist, I learn by doing. Each client and professional consultation provides me with opportunities to create practical programs and techniques for older adults with cognitive impairment. It is in this manner that I present my views of therapeutic, strength-based interventions for adults with Alzheimer's disease. The goal of all therapeutic intervention is to engage a person with dementia in life experiences for as long as possible. This book offers practical intervention practices that nurture the spirit and enhance the quality of life for individuals dealing with chronic cognitive and memory losses. It is my mission to share with family members, caregivers, and geriatric practitioners the activities and environmental modifications that promote meaningful and joyful interactions for adults with dementia.

People with Alzheimer's and other progressive dementias experience opportunities for social and emotional interactions throughout the duration of the disease. In most instances the ability to communicate diminishes before an individual loses the ability to feel. Adults in the later stages of dementia still have feelings. Lacking vocabulary, they communicate emotions by crying, yelling, touching, looking, and smiling. These expressions are windows of opportunity for elder care professionals and family members to connect with an individual. Geriatric professionals and caregivers require strategies and tools to discover these unique windows of opportunity for each person. Individualized and strength-based programming offers practitioners the necessary tools to develop appropriate and enjoyable activities for people with dementia to nurture the spirit and maintain quality of life for as long as possible and is a positive approach to therapeutic intervention. These activities do more than take up time. They are meaningful and life-enhancing experiences because they are based on the person's remaining strengths, abilities, and preferences.

Geriatric care practitioners, including recreational therapists, social workers, psychologists, speech-language pathologists, physical therapists, occupational therapists, dance therapists, music therapists, and nurses, know *why* people with dementias need recreational activities. However, knowing how to select specific activities for an individual creates challenges. Are all recreational activities appropriate for every individual? Should all individuals participate in music, dance, and crafts activities? The answer, of course, is no. Individualized, strength-based activities emphasize a person's previous interests and talents as well as current capabilities.

This book provides a framework for selecting and modifying activities based on what an individual enjoys and can still do. This positive approach emphasizes a person's unique interests and remaining competencies. By focusing on activities that highlight what an individual with dementia can still do and enjoy, practitioners and family members are ensuring that the person has opportunities to engage in life for as long as possible.

In The Ethicist section of *The New York Times Magazine*, an anonymous person wrote

My mother has been having memory issues for a number of years. Her neurologist has been telling her it is "mild dementia." Her cognitive impairment and memory loss have worsened and I recently met the neurologist without her. He told me that she has Alzheimer's. He felt we should not yet tell my mother, as that diagnosis has been her greatest fear and it would be too devastating. He felt we could not tell my father unless we told my mother. I am uncomfortable keeping this terrible secret. Is it better to tell a loved one of the prognosis they fear, or is it more ethical to let them live in hopes that they have escaped it?

Chuck Klosterman, the essayist, responded

The fact that Alzheimer's is your mom's greatest fear validates just how essential those faculties are to the quality of her life; it's possible she views the onset of Alzheimer's to be a version of living death. This being the case, the dilemma must be viewed in the context of dying. If your mother had terminal cancer, would you hide that news from her? I assume you would not. You would want her to have the opportunity to initiate final, meaningful conversations with the people she values most. You would want her to have a chance to cogently look back at the life she has already lived. (Klosterman, 2012, To Tell or Not to Tell [June 24])

I agree with Klosterman's response. Instead of concealing the diagnosis of Alzheimer's from the mother, both the mother and her family members need to come together and find ways to enable this woman to continue to have meaningful interactions with her loved ones throughout the duration of her illness. This is what needs to be done. The question, however, is how best can the mother, her family, and her caregivers address the effects of the disease over time? This book provides answers and, in turn, offers an optimistic approach to a pessimistic diagnosis.

Introduction

This book provides those who care for adults with Alzheimer's disease and related dementias with a framework for engaging and communicating with these individuals while preserving their dignity and respecting their needs and choices. Such considerations are based on a reasoned examination of a person's life history and current interests and needs, and the development of activities that match a person's interests and strengths. This approach is also based on a multiple intelligence model, which provides a framework for choosing activities based on what a person enjoys and can still do. All leisure activities are deliberate and carefully selected to suit an individual's preferences and current skills. The goal of this individualized approach is to enable the adult with dementia to maintain a sense of well-being and to experience personal joy.

Two dominant themes of many of the different approaches to providing care for people with Alzheimer's are keeping individuals active and helping them feel productive (Kalb, 2000). These themes are the underlying principles of the activities in this book, as demonstrated through several key features of the outlined approach. First, the overall philosophy of the approach is based on the recognition of the importance of an individual's past, present, and future context. A second feature is the emphasis on assessment, specifically a systematic assessment, to effectively plan activities. One of the major components is the multidimensional assessment process that provides valuable planning information from three different perspectives: staff, family, and the individual. Another key component of the assessment process, and one that supports the goals of keeping individuals active and productive, is a method for identifying a person's strengths and abilities, based on Howard Gardner's multiple intelligence model (1983, 1993). Information derived from the assessments can then be used by staff or family members to match activities to a person's previous and current interests based on his or her remaining strengths and abilities, thereby engaging the individual and enhancing his or her feelings of self-worth.

About the Book

The strength-based approach outlined in this book includes three comprehensive assessment tools that enable both professionals and family members to understand why certain activities are more appropriate than others for someone with dementia, to match activities to a person's waning abilities, and to engage the individual in positive and meaningful experiences at any stage in the progression of the disease. These informal observation inventories include the Informal Geriatric Strength-Based Inventory, the Caregiver Questionnaire and Checklist, and the Personal Preferences Inventory. When all three have been completed, a Strength-Based Summary Sheet is then used to provide practitioners with the necessary framework for appraising the unique remaining capabilities of each individual living with the diagnosis of a progressive dementia. The completed summary is the means for devising an individualized care plan. A fourth informal observation tool, the Simplified Inventory of Multiple Potential and Leisure Engagement, or the SIMPLE, is a quick and easy-to-use questionnaire for both family members and caregivers to assess the current competencies of a person with mild dementia and to enable those who are involved in caring for the person to plan activities accordingly.

Chapter 1 discusses the theoretical model for and goals of strength-based programming for individuals with Alzheimer's disease and other dementias, including the rationale for using this intervention in geriatric activity planning. Chapter 2 details how each of the four assessment tools is to be used, including the information gleaned from each and recommendations for communicating the information to family and staff members. Successful communication among key people is essential in any type of care planning. Two guides, the Dementia Care Staff Guide and the Memory Loss Caregiver Guide, are provided to assist with this critical element. Three case studies at the end of Chapter 2 show how each of the assessment tools and guides should be used. Chapters 3, 4, and 5 are devoted to strength-based practices. Providing meaningful activities to adults with a progressive dementia that they still can do and enjoy is the primary focus of all leisure experiences. In Chapter 3, readers are offered examples of how to offer leisure activities in a unique reverse developmental sequence, meaning from complex to simple. Comprehensive lists of strength-based activities are organized according to the three phases of dementia (mild, moderate, severe), as well as by which strengths and abilities the person possesses (based on Gardner's multiple intelligence model). Modifying activities and materials to correspond with an individual's waning cognitive and memory skills is a crucial aspect of strength-based programming. In Chapter 4, Michelle Bourgeois provides vital information on how to adapt tasks and activities to match an individual's strengths and preferences with his or her remaining abilities. Knowing how to adapt activities of personal interest allows the person to remain engaged and feel productive. In Chapter 5, Joan Green describes many new roles for technology in strength-based programming and offers many suggestions of devices, online sites, computer software, and other technological resources that aid individuals with memory and cognitive loss.

Communication is an important aspect of a strength-based intervention. Chapter 6 offers several individual lists of practical tips, each with a specific intent, to facilitate communication with a person with dementia and to help both family members and professionals engage in pleasant conversations and experiences with the individual, whether the person is living at home or residing in a long-term care facility. Individuals with cognitive loss might not remember what was said, but they tend to remember how they felt. It is the feeling of well-being and relating to another person that nurtures the spirit and maintains one's interest in life. Author Jolene Brackey refers to this positive approach as creating "moments of joy" for someone who has dementia.

Another feature of this book that contributes to the themes of engagement and productivity is the compilation of resources contained in the appendixes. Of particular note is the list of books available to use with children to help them understand dementia, which can be mysterious and confusing for them.

———————

Issues of quality of life arise throughout life. It seems, however, that only at certain times are quality-of-life issues magnified. One of these times is as people age and change due to various health reasons. Unfortunately, too little attention has been given to quality-of-life issues as they affect older adults with Alzheimer's disease. The approach outlined in this book contributes to the efforts to raise awareness about maintaining quality of life throughout the progression of dementia. As stated in the Preface, the purpose of this book is to provide positive options to a pessimistic situation. The practical framework and activities offered throughout are aimed at enriching the lives of adults with Alzheimer's disease. The individualized strength-based approach provides family members and practitioners with a useful resource for identifying activities that a person with dementia can do successfully. Most important, the activities are individualized (based on individual interests and strengths), which can enhance feelings of personal fulfillment and satisfaction as well as a sense of productivity.

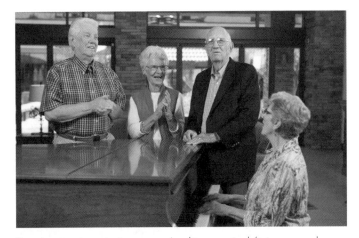

Participating in a singing group (auditory-musical/interpersonal strengths)

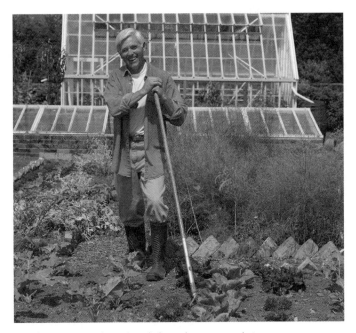

Gardening (naturalistic/tactile-kinesthetic strengths)

Chapter 1

Introduction to Strength-Based Programming

What do a diverse group of celebrities such as singer Perry Como, President Ronald Reagan, boxer Sugar Ray Robinson, abstract expressionist William DeKooning, theater and film director Otto Preminger, Senator Barry Goldwater, chef Joyce Chen, actor Charlton Heston, and painter Norman Rockwell have in common? They lived with and later died from Alzheimer's disease. In 2012 in the United States alone, Alzheimer's disease and related dementias affected approximately 5.4 million individuals and is the sixth-leading cause of death. According to the *Alzheimer's Disease Facts and Figures* report, 1 in 8 Americans aged 65 and older has Alzheimer's, and nearly half of people aged 85 and older have the disease (Alzheimer's Association, 2012). The report further estimates that by 2050 up to 16 million people will have the disease. On average, Alzheimer's disease lasts about 8 years, although it may last as little as 2 years or as long as 20 years.

According to the Alzheimer's Association, *dementia* is a general term for loss of memory and other mental abilities severe enough to interfere with daily life. It is caused by physical changes in the brain. Alzheimer's disease is the most common type of dementia, accounting for 60 to 80 percent of cases. Other neurodegenerative causes of dementia include vascular dementia, dementia with Lewy bodies (DLB), Parkinson's disease, Creutzfeldt-Jakob disease, Huntington's disease, Pick's disease, and Korsakoff syndrome. In this book, the terms *Alzheimer's disease (Alzheimer's)*, *dementia*, and *neurodegenerative dementia* will be used to describe a progressive dementia. Although currently drug treatments exist that may temporarily improve symptoms, there is no cure. "The only certainty," one individual in the mild phase of Alzheimer's describes, "is I'm losing my personality and becoming a nothing." This is the harsh reality of all dementias.

And yet there is much that can be done to support the person over the course of the disease and maximize his or her quality of life. A positive and effective approach to therapeutic intervention for people with neurological dementias is strength-based programming. Just as the optimist views a glass as half full instead of half empty, a strength-based approach emphasizes an individual's remaining competencies, not his or her disabilities. Strength-based practices accentuate what an individual still can do, while cautioning individuals against pursuing tasks that are too complex and dangerous, such as operating a car. Currently, it is customary to diagnose neurodegenerative diseases based on what individuals no longer can do. The Informal Geriatric Strength-Based Inventory (IGSI), which is discussed in Chapter 2, turns this approach on its head and enables professionals working with older adults to validate each individual's current performance level in terms of what the person *can* do and then individualize appropriate activities matched to his or her abilities during the mild, moderate, and severe phases of this progressive disease (Eisner, 2001). Likewise, the SIMPLE, also discussed in Chapter 2, enables family members and caregivers to quickly assess the individual at home.

The goal of strength-based programming is to assist individuals with neurodegenerative dementias to maintain a quality of life for as long as possible. Rather than merely occupying time, carefully individualized leisure and recreational activities encourage socialization, prompt recall, and maintain an individual's interest in life. All individualized, strength-based activities fuse activity and communication therapy into the daily routines of people with Alzheimer's. Individualizing intervention enables geriatric care professionals to meet the unique capabilities and needs of affected older adults. This, in turn, helps increase the number of opportunities that an individual can still enjoy. Although a person with dementia might not recall what he or she did, the person seems to retain how he or she felt when engaged in a positive experience.

Progression of Dementia

Understanding the progressive phases associated with a neurodegenerative dementia is the first step toward creating appropriate leisure activities. As a neurodegenerative disease evolves, patients become more and more limited in the activities they can do. Practitioners and caregivers, planning meaningful activities for adults with Alzheimer's disease and related dementias, must anticipate how the progression of the disease affects an individual's ability to perform tasks. To successfully engage patients in meaningful interactions throughout the duration of their illnesses, activities must be gradually modified and adapted to coordinate with an individual's diminishing cognition, communication, and memory.

Alzheimer's disease and related progressive dementias progress in fairly predictable phases. Barry Reisberg, M.D., clinical director of the New York

University School of Medicine's Silberstein Aging and Dementia Research Center, developed the Global Deterioration Scale (GDS) and Functional Assessment Staging Tool (FAST) (Reisberg, Ferris, de Leon & Crook, 1982; Reisberg, 1988). This widely used assessment, based on Reisberg's theory of retrogenesis, provides a general idea of how abilities change during the course of the disease. Reisberg's concept of retrogenesis describes a progressive reversal of developmental stages in a person and is summarized as follows:

1. The Mild or Forgetful Phase (Stages 1 and 2) corresponds to normal human development from 14 years of age to adulthood. In this phase of dementia individuals suffer no subjective or objective changes in intellectual functioning.

2. The Moderate or Confused Phase (Stages 3, 4, and 5) corresponds to normal human development from 8 to 13 years of age. Individuals with dementia progress in these stages from normal age-related forgetfulness to losing the ability to handle daily routines, such as shopping, driving a vehicle, managing household finances, and finally losing the ability to live alone.

3. The Severe or Confused Phase (Stages 6 and 7) corresponds to normal human development from infancy to 7 years of age. Individuals in this phase progress from requiring assistance in basic self-help and toileting tasks to losing the abilities to walk and talk. During this final stage of dementia, the individual falls into a stupor or coma and eventually dies.

Using Reisberg's assessments enables practitioners, caregivers, and family members to establish realistic expectations as well as a common-sense approach to Alzheimer's care. For example, practitioners attempting to determine the appropriateness of a phase II patient operating a vehicle can consider the question in the context of imagining the suitability of a 13-year-old driving a car. Likewise, to fully comprehend the capabilities of an early phase III patient, practitioners and caregivers could refer to the characteristics of a 7-year-old. Would parents leave a 7-year-old at home alone? Of course not. Should a caregiver leave an adult who functions at a 7-year-old level alone? Of course not. Understanding Reisberg's three phases of dementia provides caregivers with solutions to dilemmas concerning the care and supervision of an individual throughout the progressive phases of a neurodegenerative disease.

Strength-Based Programming

A strength-based program for individuals with cognitive and memory loss is a *can-do* approach to maintaining one's quality of life throughout the duration of the dementia. More than simply occupying leisure time, strength-based geriatric programming provides individuals with ongoing and meaningful activities, prompts communication, and assists them in engaging in social interactions for as long as possible. As the disease progresses from the mild, moderate, to the severe phase, activities are modified in a systematic manner, thus prompting the individual to respond, react, and communicate at his or her greatest (even if limited) potential.

Strength-based programming provides geriatric care professionals with a framework for selecting materials and activities as well as accountability to the therapeutic process by offering a clear-cut rationale for every recreational activity and intervention program. Should all individuals be required to participate in every group activity? The answer is no. Professionals use a strength-based framework to select activities based on an individual's previous interests and current capabilities.

Rationale for Strength-Based Programming

Educational principles and practices developed for children with learning challenges are rich resources for creating programs for older adults with cognitive and memory impairment. Difficulties with initiating and anticipating events are common to both older adults and children with cognitive impairment. As dementia progresses, the older adult eventually loses the ability to initiate actions and anticipate actions. Education professionals handle this same impairment in children by teaching to a child's unique learning style. Teachers use a learning style method to teach children new concepts, while geriatric practitioners use the learning style approach—strength-based programming—to stimulate long-term memory and engagement.

Evidence shows that educational strategies may be adapted to meet the needs of adults with cognitive impairment. Independent studies by Camp and colleagues (1997) and Dreher (1997) describe successful adaptations of Montessori teaching methods. Dreher states that "action without a purpose fatigues," and that people with Alzheimer's often suffer through endless, aimless activity. Activities that resemble useful work from the person's past, however, spark an older adult's attention. Montessori-based dementia programming focuses on working with the strengths and abilities that remain, finding the person behind the memory problems, and engaging the individual to promote feelings of well-being (Joltin, 2005). Likewise, Linda Levine Madori's Therapeutic Thematic Arts Programming method (TTAP Method) combines therapeutic recreation with the creative arts using a framework based on the cognitive developmental theories of Jean Piaget, Benjamin Bloom, and Howard Gardner. In her work as an art and recreation therapist, Levine Madori has incorporated into thematic programming current research on brain functioning as well as the basic principles of multiple intelligence as the bases to facilitate learning, boost memory, encourage the use of language, and enhance socialization for those with dementia. TTAP Method programming allows for infinite variations on themes based on the personal interests and individual strengths of each participant at each stage of the disease progression.

Theoretical Model for Strength-Based Programming

Strength-based programming draws from Howard Gardner's theory of multiple intelligences to individualize activities for heterogeneous groupings of older adults with varying levels of cognitive and communication skills. Gardner, a psychologist at the Harvard Graduate School of Education, developed a theory of intelligence that led away from what he called the "IQ way of thinking" developed by Lewis Terman (1916). Gardner notes that when intelligence tests were first used during World War I, they were a means to categorize people, especially the soldiers, based on various competencies. In his influential book *Frames of Mind* (1983), Gardner rebuts Terman's IQ theory with the theory of multiple intelligences. Gardner initially introduced the following seven intelligences:

> verbal-linguistic
> logical-mathematical
> visual-spatial
> tactile-kinesthetic
> auditory-musical
> interpersonal
> intrapersonal

He later introduced an eighth, naturalistic intelligence, followed by existential intelligence (Gardner, 1999). See Figure 1.1 for a diagram of the types of multiple intelligences.

According to Gardner,

- Individuals with strong **verbal-linguistic** talents are usually attracted to activities involving listening, speaking, reading, and writing.

- Individuals having **logical-mathematical** strengths excel at tasks involving numbers, patterns, logical reasoning, and order.

- Individuals with strong **visual-spatial** intelligence normally excel at activities involving seeing and doing, such as drawing, building, designing, and creating visual images.

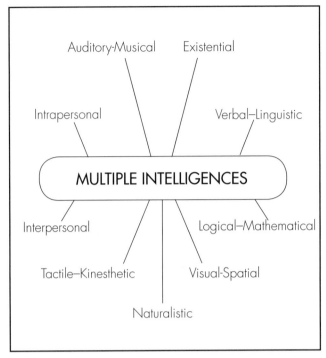

Figure 1.1. Diagram of the types of multiple intelligences.

- Individuals with outstanding **tactile-kinesthetic** talents may be good with their hands and/or possess exceptional physical dexterity. They may be drawn to activities that involve physical movement, such as sports or using their hands to create objects.

- People possessing extraordinary **auditory-musical** intelligence have "an excellent ear" for words, music, and languages.

- Individuals with heightened **interpersonal** intelligence are "people persons" and usually perform best in social and group situations.

- Individuals possessing keen **intrapersonal** aptitude "know themselves." They enjoy working alone and have a heightened sense of self-esteem, intuition, and individualism. People who have exceptional intrapersonal intelligence may be attracted to professions involving philosophy, visual arts, research, and entrepreneurship.

- Individuals with strong **naturalistic** talents are "in tune with nature." They usually are drawn to occupations such as animal training, fishing, natural and animal sciences, and landscaping.

- Individuals with strong **existential** intelligence usually are keenly interested in life's great questions involving religion, philosophy, and ethics.

Due to the severe and progressive nature of a neurodegenerative disease, existential intelligence has not been considered as a possible area of remaining competency. O lder adults who have severe memory and cognitive impairments eventually lose the ability to comprehend and discuss existential questions.

The way to recognize remaining strengths is by observing an individual's behaviors. For a comprehensive listing of behaviors associated with each area of intelligence and represented in a reverse developmental order (from complex to simple tasks), as per Reisberg's theory of retrogenesis, see Appendix A.

Gardner (1983) maintains that matching an individual's job or avocation with his or her natural intelligence enables the person to realize his or her full potential. Likewise, strength-based programming uses a multiple intelligence framework to match all interactions and activities with an older adult's remaining capabilities, thus enabling the person with Alzheimer's to participate in life at his or her fullest potential for as long as possible. In his book, *Multiple Intelligences: The Theory in Practice* (1993), Gardner briefly applies his theory to dementia. He notes that

> Alzheimer's disease, a form of presenile dementia, appears to attack posterior brain zones with a special ferocity, leaving spatial, logical, and linguistic computations severely impaired. Yet, Alzheimer's patients will often remain well groomed, socially proper, and continually apologetic for their errors. In contrast, Pick's disease, another variety of presenile dementia that is more frontally oriented, entails a rapid loss of social graces." (p. 23)

Recognizing Strengths in Geriatric Populations

Strength-based programming adapts multiple intelligence theory to geriatric activity planning. A multiple intelligence model provides a framework for geriatric care professionals to discover an individual's remaining competencies and preferences and to develop meaningful and successful interventions. Table 1.1 provides an overview of the skills and activities associated with each area of intelligence. The reader should be mindful that activities listed in column four ("Benefits from") may not be appropriate for all individuals with dementia, especially those with severe dementia. Comprehensive information on providing appropriate strength-based intervention throughout the progression of a neurodegenerative disease is provided in Chapter 3.

When individuals are aware of their deficiencies, geriatric care professionals must accentuate remaining competencies. Patients need to discover what they still can do and enjoy. For example, a 75-year-old woman with moderate stage dementia said to her daughter, "I will not go back to the neurologist. All

Table 1.1. Overview of strength-based programming for adults with Alzheimer's disease and related progressive neurological dementias

Area of remaining intelligence	Previously was good at:	May like to:	Benefits from:
Verbal–Linguistic	Telling stories, giving speeches, creative writing, word games	Read, write, and participate in group discussions	Activities involving listening, speaking, reading, and writing
Mathematical–Logical	Math, reasoning, logical and analytical tasks, problem solving	Know the rules of games; work with numbers; keep score of group games and ask questions	Keeping to a time schedule; playing board games and cards; working with the computer; working with math problems; and sorting and organizing objects
Visual–Spatial	Visualizing images and concepts; using maps and charts; completing jigsaw puzzles and mazes; reading; drawing	Draw, build, and create things; look at pictures; watch TV	Using visual cues (posters, pictures, bulletin board displays, signs); working with colors, shapes, and textures; art activities and possibly computer games
Auditory–Musical	Listening and speaking; music appreciation and perhaps singing and/ or playing musical instruments; speaking more than one language; rhymes, riddles, and poems; noticing changes in pitch tone and volume	Listen to music; participate in sing-alongs; play a musical instrument; move and sway to music; listen to others speak	Music and dance activities; using auditory or verbal cues to recall information; singing, playing musical instruments; watching musicals on TV
Tactile–Kinesthetic	Physical activities; exercise classes; dancing; hiking/ walking; using hands to construct or create	Move around, touch, and talk; use gestures and body language to express thoughts	Physical exercise and art activities involving touch, movement, and interacting with space (use blocks and objects); using hands-on materials, such as clay and yarn, to stimulate recall
Interpersonal	Understanding people; leading others; organizing social functions; participating in community and group activities	Be with people; talk to others; participate in social and group activities	Participating in group discussions and support groups; sharing, comparing, relating, and reminiscing with others
Intrapersonal	Understanding the self; focusing inward; following instincts and intuition; being original; pursing own personal goals	Work alone and at own pace; pursue own interests; work on own personal projects	Individual counseling sessions; self-paced activities; having own physical space; individualized and personalized projects and activities
Naturalistic	Gardening; hiking; animal and plant care; natural sciences	Be outdoors; sit near the window; care for animals and pets	Interacting with nature; gardening activities; looking at pictures, movies, and TV shows that focus on animals and nature; being outdoors

the doctor makes me do is answer questions. I can't do it, and I refuse to be humiliated again. I might have memory problems, but all the doctor does is remind me of what I can't do." The daughter, aware of her mother's intrapersonal skills, responded: "How would you feel if the doctor said your mathematical and short-term memory skills are weak, but your insight and intuition are excellent?" The mother replied, "Not so bad."

The daughter proceeded to list her mother's remaining competencies. She emphasized the woman's excellent intuition, sense of style, artistic awareness, sensitivity, and ability to express happiness and love. She then shared the list with her mother. Hearing a list of her personal characteristics, the mother smiled and said, "Bless you. I feel better already." Individuals who have dementia might forget what has been said to them, but they tend to recall how they felt about a particular interaction. Successfully reminding a person of what he or she still can do fosters feelings of well-being.

When evaluating the remaining capabilities of an Alzheimer's patient, professionals must consider various factors, such as the individual's great passion in life, his or her previous occupation, and his or her previous lifestyle. They must recognize that an individual might have had multiple interests and talents. For example, a patient may have been a journalist whose hobby was tennis. In the early phase of dementia, this individual would most likely exhibit an interest in and propensity for verbal-linguistic (journalist) as well as tactile-kinesthetic (tennis) activities. As the disease progresses, and the person's skill level changes, ongoing assessments are required to determine if these two areas are still remaining strengths, and, if so, how activities can be adapted to allow the individual to continue to enjoy and connect with his or her past interests.

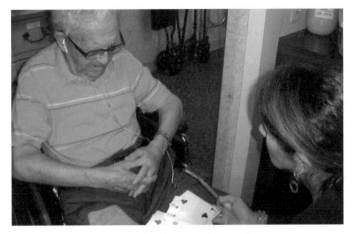

Playing card games (logical-mathematical strength)

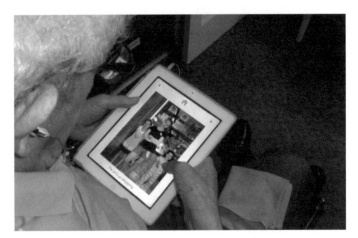

Viewing family pictures via a mobile tablet (verbal-linguistic/intrapersonal strengths)

Chapter 2

Assessing the Potential of Adults with Cognitive and Memory Loss

In her book, *Therapeutic Thematic Arts Programming for Older Adults*, Linda Levine Madori states that "each person has different strengths and weaknesses, which requires the therapist to create programming for all levels of functioning within the group. This is one of the most complex tasks for therapists, yet they rarely are trained to handle these situations." (Levine Madori, 2007, p. 23) Levine Madori's Therapeutic Thematic Arts Programming method (TTAP Method), a strength-based intervention, assists the therapist in meeting the needs of an individual with Alzheimer's disease or other dementia by first assessing which of Gardner's seven learning styles he or she still retains in the face of cognitive and memory loss. This chapter discusses the "how to" of assessing and translating the behaviors of an individual with Alzheimer's into a multiple intelligence framework through the use of comprehensive assessment tools. A more simplified assessment alternative, the SIMPLE, is also included. Three case study examples at the end of the chapter illustrate how to use each tool.

The Assessment Process

An essential component of addressing the needs of adults with cognitive and memory loss is the ability to assess their former strengths and interests within the context of their present status. Assessment implies the gathering of information relative to these predetermined purposes. The formats of various successful assessment instruments (Brown & Hammill, 1990; Clark & Patton, 1997; Conners, 1997) have influenced the design of a set of instruments described in this book that provide different perspectives of a person's former and current strengths. This assessment process includes information from the following three sources:

1. The practitioner form, known as the Informal Geriatric Strength-Based Inventory (IGSI), is completed by a staff member or other service provider who is familiar with the individual and who can respond to a series of items based on observations and experiences in working with the individual.

2. The Caregiver Questionnaire and Checklist is completed by a family member or friend who has known the individual for a significant period of time.

3. The Personal Preferences Inventory is completed by the individual. Asking a person to complete this form may not always be appropriate, because it will depend largely on the individual's stage of dementia, along with his or her motivation to complete it.

Once all three of these forms are completed, a comprehensive picture of a person's past and current strengths and interests becomes available to all parties. Even if only one of the forms is completed, valuable information has been obtained. These forms serve to unite practitioners from different disciplines with a shared vision of a patient's previous interests and current capabilities. Ultimately, the information that is gleaned from this process can and should be used to create care plans, the best care environments, and activities programming for persons who are experiencing cognitive and memory challenges in their everyday lives. To assist practitioners with these goals, the Strength-Based Summary Sheet was developed as a tool to help summarize the pertinent information that emerges from the assessment process.

Using the set of three instruments, professionals get measurable results that correlate with the Minimum Data Set (MDS). The MDS is part of the U.S. federally mandated process for clinical assessment of all residents in Medicare or Medicaid certified nursing homes. The MDS process is a medically-based assessment of each resident's functional capabilities. The IGSI provides measurable results of patterns related to the cognitive, communication and hearing, mood and behavior, psychosocial well-being, and activity pursuit sections of the MDS. Practitioners who are familiar with the IGSI will find that it simplifies the task of completing the MDS.

The Dementia Care Staff Guide (for use in a residential care facility) and the Memory Loss Caregiver Guide (for use at home) both simplify the results of the strength-based assessment by providing family members, caregivers, and practitioners with straightforward information on how to speak with, pacify, and persuade an individual with Alzheimer's. (All three assessment tools as well as the two guides are available for free download at http://www.healthpropress. com/eisner/34snEi03f.) These personalized forms assure that all of whom are caring for an older adult with Alzheimer's are aware of and make use of the same strength-based procedures. The Dementia Care Staff Guide may also include key aspects of a resident's care plan.

Informal Geriatric Strength-Based Inventory

The Informal Geriatric Strength-Based Inventory (IGSI) is a comprehensive assessment instrument to determine an individual's current abilities and interests and is completed by one or more practitioners who have direct and regular contact with the individual.

The IGSI is divided into the following three sections:

- Section 1: Collects background information about the individual. This section is straightforward and should not be difficult for the practitioner to complete.

- Section 2: Requires the practitioner to rate the competency of the individual on 80 items that are organized into 8 categories related to the various areas of intelligence identified by Gardner (1993):

  Area I: Linguistic-Verbal
  Area II: Logical-Mathematical
  Area III: Visual-Spatial
  Area IV: Tactile-Kinesthetic
  Area V: Auditory-Musical
  Area VI: Interpersonal
  Area VII: Intrapersonal
  Area VIII: Naturalistic

The practitioner completing the form has six rating choices for each item. The response options are as follow:

  NA = Not applicable. To be used when the item does not apply to the individual.
  0 = Never. Indicates that the person does not show the behavior at all, even though opportunities have arisen when the behavior could have been displayed.
  1 = Seldom. Indicates that the person shows the behavior on an infrequent basis.
  2 = Frequently. Indicates that the person shows the behavior on a regular basis.
  3 = Always. To be used when the person shows the behavior whenever given the opportunity to do so.
  ? = Don't know. To be used when the informant does not know whether the individual displays the behavior.

The next step of determining the areas of strength for the individual is to total the number of rating points for each intelligence area. The ratings for each area are totaled and recorded in the Total Score box. This process is illustrated in case study #1 (pp. 24–33), which uses the Verbal-Linguistic intelligence area as an example.

In section 2 of the IGSI, space is also provided after each intelligence area to list any additional comments that may be pertinent to the ratings, such as other information that relates to the category but is not addressed by any of the items in the inventory.

Section 3: Provides a summary of the competency areas. This form is completed by transferring the total scores for each intelligence in section 2 to the appropriate line in the Summary of Competency Areas section.

Once these totals are recorded, circle the areas with the most points, then rank them in order in the spaces provided. The area with the most points indicates the area of greatest remaining competency. Later, this information will be transferred to the Strength-Based Summary Sheet.

Caregiver Questionnaire and Checklist

Although the Caregiver Questionnaire and Checklist is designed to be completed by a family member, the form could also be filled in by a friend or other close acquaintance. The person who completes this form, however, must have known the individual for a significant period of time and currently be very familiar with the person. Case study #1 (pp. 34–40) and case study #2 (pp. 66–72) show sample pages of the instrument.

This assessment contains the following three sections:

Section 1: Requests a few basic descriptive responses about the individual and the caregiver.
Section 2: Includes 17 open-ended questions related to the individual's former and current abilities and interests.
Section 3: Provides space to check off activities that the individual currently does.

The results derived from this assessment should be summarized in narrative form and incorporated into the Strength-Based Summary Sheet. The information provided by caregivers is valuable because it provides a rich context for understanding an individual's past and present based on the perceptions of someone who knows the individual well.

Personal Preferences Inventory

The Personal Preferences Inventory is important because it represents the personal sentiments of the individual. This instrument requires that the individual be able to communicate his or her feelings about the items being presented. Furthermore, an assumption is made that an individual's responses represent his or her true feelings. Sample pages for how to use the Personal Preferences Inventory are shown in case study #1 (pp. 41–50) and case study #2 (pp. 73–82).

The inventory is divided into the following four sections:

Section 1: Collects basic information about the individual

Section 2: Features five general, open-ended questions regarding personal preferences

Section 3: Used to rate a patient's likes and dislikes, much like section 2 of the IGSI

Section 4: Presents summary information

Section 3, being the most comprehensive section, is organized according to the various intelligence areas and includes 80 items. The individual reacts to each item by indicating his or her level of interest in engaging in the listed activity. The rating scale includes the following options:

0 = Strongly dislike. Indicates that the person does not like the activity at all.

1 = Do not like. Indicates that the person does not care for the activity but might do it on occasion.

2 = Like. Indicates that the person somewhat likes to engage in the activity.

3 = Like very much. Indicates that the person very much enjoys the activity and would probably engage in it often if given the opportunity.

? = Don't know. To be used when the individual does not know whether he or she likes the activity. Such a response might indicate never having been exposed to the activity.

To determine which of the areas an individual likes, it is necessary to total the number of rating points for each intelligence area. To do this, add the ratings for each item and then record the number in the Total Score box. At the end of the inventory, the total score for each intelligence area should be transferred to the appropriate line in section 4 of the inventory, the summary of likes and dislikes. Once these totals are recorded, circle the areas with the most points, then rank these in order in the spaces provided. The area with the most points indicates the area that the individual likes the most. Later, this information will be transferred to the Strength-Based Summary Sheet, which is discussed in the next section. As is common to all of the forms presented in this book, space is provided after each intelligence area to write any additional notes.

Strength-Based Summary Sheet

The Strength-Based Summary Sheet requires the practitioner to summarize the information collected during the assessment process. Although the person responsible for completing this summary sheet might vary depending on the setting in which the individual with cognitive and memory loss is located, the person completing the form is typically a practitioner who is familiar with the individual. By summarizing information obtained from the various sources, this document can assist practitioners in designing interventions that are based on the strengths and interests of the individual. Case study #1 (pp. 51–52) and case study #2 (pp. 83–84) display how the tool can be used.

The Strength-Based Summary Sheet is composed of three sections. The first section provides space to write the person's name and the date when the form was completed. The date is important, as interests, and particularly competencies, can change over time. The second section contains space to record the summary information from the three forms. The total scores from the IGSI and the Personal Preferences Inventory are recorded in their respective columns. Information from the Caregiver Questionnaire and Checklist can be recorded in the "Caregiver Checklist" column. The depth of information that can be recorded here is at the discretion of the person completing the summary sheet; often, simply placing a check in these columns is sufficient. Finally, check marks are placed in the last column to indicate the areas of strength. Section 3 of the Strength-Based Summary Sheet organizes the findings by prioritizing the areas of strength.

Communicating the Results of a Strength-Based Assessment

Communication is the key to intervention. The success of a strength-based assessment depends on how effectively practitioners communicate the findings to those practitioners who interact directly with the cognitively impaired individual. The usefulness of the assessment depends on the implementation and integration of strength-based intervention into the environment and daily routines of the patient. A successful intervention program occurs when those individuals involved in the therapeutic process incorporate a patient's remaining strengths on a daily, or even hourly, basis. The Dementia Care Staff Guide and Memory Loss Caregiver Guide are two methods by which to communicate the assessment findings.

The Dementia Care Staff Guide (p. 22) is designed for staff members who work in a day center, residential assisted living, or long-term care facility. This brief form may be an integral component of a care plan. Staff members can jointly complete this page, guaranteeing that each staff member has a clear understanding of an individual's strengths and weaknesses. Furthermore, the form assures that all staff members use the same strategies when working with a particular individual. Once the Dementia Care Staff Guide has been completed, it should be displayed in a convenient, visible location. Practitioners may choose to put it on a staff bulletin board and in an activity plan book, as well as in the individual's medical or personal file. Case study #1 (p. 53) displays how the Dementia Care Staff Guide can be used.

The Memory Loss Caregiver Guide (p. 21) is a brief form for family members and caregivers. This guide uses the term *memory loss* instead of *Alzheimer's disease* or *dementia* because family members and patients may be overly sensitive to these labels. At times, verbal instructions or lengthy medical reports are too challenging for those trying to cope with the progressive disease of a loved one. The Memory Loss Caregiver Guide simplifies communication by highlighting the most significant information and practical suggestions. This form pinpoints what the person still can do, which intervention will diminish agitation, and who to call in case of an emergency. This written form may be laminated and attached to the kitchen refrigerator or family message center. Caregivers are urged to photocopy this guide and place it in other rooms, such as the bathroom, bedroom, and living room. In addition, this guide enhances communication between professional caregivers and family members, thus promoting consistency in patient care. Case study #1 (p. 54) and case study #2 (p. 85) are examples of how the Memory Loss Caregiver Guide can be used.

At the top of both the Dementia Care Staff Guide and the Memory Loss Caregiver Guide is the reminder to "avoid verbal disagreements" in bold. Verbal disagreements create agitation for the patient as well as stress for the caregiver. Agreeing with the patient or changing the subject or environment enables caregivers to gently guide the individual toward a more harmonious interaction. For example, when patients with more moderate or severe dementia are agitated, they usually call out for a loved one, such as a father. When this happens, do not tell the person that his or her loved one is not available or is dead. Calm the individual by gently asking him or her about the loved one. You might say, "Your father was a wonderful person. What's his name? What did you and your dad do together?" Eventually a pleasant conversation will replace the person's overwhelming need for comfort.

The SIMPLE

Finally, the Simple Inventory of Multiple Potential and Leisure Engagement (SIMPLE) is a quick-and-easy evaluation that family members, at-home caregivers, and professionals, when faced with time constraints, can use to assess an individual's current capabilities. It allows users to gain a brief multiple-intelligence overview of an individual's strengths and weaknesses. Using the SIMPLE with a loved one who has mild dementia provides family members with valuable information in understanding their loved one's current status and enables all who are involved in caring for the person to incorporate his or her remaining strengths while also recognizing the individual's diminished abilities. It is recommended that professionals use the three comprehensive strength-based inventories for all initial evaluations, and then use the SIMPLE as a follow-up reassessment tool to evaluate an individual's changing capabilities throughout the duration of the disease. Furthermore, the results of the SIMPLE may also be used to complete the Memory Loss Caregiver Guide. (The SIMPLE is available for free download at http://www.healthpropress. com/eisner/34snEi03f.)

Case Studies with Completed Assessments and Communication Guides

The case study section that begins on page 23 includes samples of completed assessments and communication guides for three individuals. The intent of this section is threefold: (1) to illustrate how the forms should be completed; (2) to provide examples of how the information obtained from the assessments can be used to guide interventions; and (3) to demonstrate how communication guides can be used.

The SIMPLE
(Simplified Inventory of Multiple Potential and Leisure Engagement)

Section 1: Basic Information

Date: _____   Individual's name: _____

Individual's preferred name or nickname: _____

Informant's name and relation to individual: _____

Section 2: Current Competencies

Read each item carefully. Place a number 1 on the line to the right of each activity that this individual is currently interested in and is able to perform. Total the number of points in each group of activities (a–e) and place each total in the scoring section.

1. Verbal-Linguistic (speaking, reading, writing)

a. Likes to talk to others _____

b. Participates in group discussions _____

c. Enjoys reading _____

d. Enjoys activities involving writing _____

e. Does word games, such as crossword puzzle _____

Total: _____

2. Logical-Mathematical (logic and reasoning)

a. Enjoys board games and cards _____

b. Enjoys problem solving _____

c. Excels in math calculations _____

d. Good with money management _____

e. Strong sense of time and time schedules _____

Total: _____

3. Visual-Spatial (seeing and doing)

a. Very aware of design, décor, and dress _____

b. Enjoys reading _____

c. Enjoys writing _____

d. Enjoys drawing and other art activities _____

e. Enjoys watching t.v. and looking at photos _____

Total: _____

4. Tactile-Kinesthetic (body movement and sensation of touch)

a. Enjoys dancing _____

b. Enjoys exercising and walking _____

c. Enjoys doing tasks with hands
(building, sewing, fixing things) _____

d. Enjoys sports _____

e. Doesn't like to sit for a long period of time _____

Total: _____

Continued

Engaging and Communicating with People Who Have Dementia: Finding and Using Their Strengths, by Eileen Eisner. Copyright © 2013, by Health Professions Press, Inc.

Section 2: Current Competencies *Continued*

5. Auditory-Musical (listening involving pitch, tone, and rhythm)

a. Enjoys listening to music _____

b. Enjoys singing _____

c. Plays a musical instrument _____

d. Likes books on tape and listening to the radio _____

e. Speaks and/or recognizes other languages _____

Total: _____

6. Interpersonal (social, likes people)

a. Enjoys being with people _____

b. Participates in group activities _____

c. Enjoys social events and parties _____

d. Enjoys being a part of a committee or group _____

e. Sensitive to the feelings of others _____

Total: _____

7. Intrapersonal (self-knowledge, independence)

a. Likes to work alone _____

b. Has an independent personality _____

c. Likes to be a leader _____

d. Likes to talk about him- or herself _____

e. Needs to feel important _____

Total: _____

8. Naturalistic (nature)

a. Enjoys being outdoors _____

b. Enjoys gardening _____

c. Enjoys caring for indoor plants _____

d. Loves animals _____

e. Responds to books and photos of nature _____

Total: _____

Score

Place the totals from each of the 8 areas in the correct space below for that intelligence. Circle the areas with the greatest number of points.

Verbal-Linguistic: _____

Logical-Mathematical: _____

Visual-Spatial: _____

Tactile-Kinesthetic: _____

Auditory-Musical: _____

Interpersonal: _____

Intrapersonal: _____

Naturalistic: _____

List below the areas of multiple intelligence that currently rank the highest for this individual, starting with the highest score in the first space, followed by the next-lower scores in spaces 2, 3, and 4. Number 1 indicates this individual's greatest area of remaining interest and capability.

a.i.1. _____

a.i.2. _____

a.i.3. _____

a.i.4. _____

Possible Ideas and Activities: Refer to Chapters 3, 4, and 5 of this book for specific recommendations.

Engaging and Communicating with People Who Have Dementia: Finding and Using Their Strengths, by Eileen Eisner. Copyright © 2013, by Health Professions Press, Inc.

Memory Loss Caregiver Guide

▪▪▪▪▪▪▪▪▪▪▪▪▪▪▪▪▪▪▪▪▪▪▪▪▪▪▪▪▪▪▪▪▪▪▪

AVOID VERBAL DISAGREEMENTS!

No one wins when you argue with someone who has memory problems. Change the subject or change the environment.

_____'s area of strength is _____.

Use these strength-based activities daily:

1. _____

2. _____

3. _____

4. _____

5. _____

When _____ gets agitated, use the following techniques to decrease any problem behaviors:

1. _____

2. _____

3. _____

4. _____

5. _____

Avoid the following _____

_____

Give your loved one opportunities to communicate by _____

_____.

For immediate assistance and advice, call _____ at _____.

Dementia Care Staff Guide

> ### AVOID VERBAL DISAGREEMENTS!
>
> No one wins when you argue with someone who has memory problems. Change the subject or change the environment.

Patient's name _____   Room number _____

Address the individual as _____.

Circle phase of dementia: Mild

                                           Moderate

                                           Severe

To gain this individual's attention, use the following techniques

_____

_____

This individual communicates by _____.

Remaining strengths _____

Create opportunities for the individual to use these strengths by doing the following: _____

_____

When the individual is agitated, use the following procedures to calm the individual:

1. _____

2. _____

The following interactions and activities should be avoided at all times:

1. _____

2. _____

HARRIS R.

■■■■ ■■ ■■ ■■ ■■ ■■ ■■ ■■ ■■ ■■ ■■ ■■ ■■

Age: 95

Medical diagnosis: Vascular Dementia, Diabetes

Phase of dementia: Moderate to severe

Setting: Assistive Living Residence

Assessment forms used:

Informal Geriatric Strength-Based Inventory, p. 24

Caregiver Questionnaire and Checklist, p. 34

Personal Preferences Inventory, p. 41

Guides used:

Dementia Care Staff Guide, p. 53

Memory Loss Caregiver Guide, p. 54

Informal Geriatric Strength-Based Inventory

▬▬▬▬▬▬▬▬▬▬▬▬▬▬▬▬▬▬▬▬▬▬▬▬▬▬▬▬▬▬▬▬▬▬▬▬▬▬▬

Section 1: Background Information

Individual's name _Harris Rose_   Date _January, 2013_

Date of birth _12-14-18_   Age _95_

Address or residential setting room number _____ Gardens Assisted living

Suite 218

Check the appropriate boxes:

☐ Living at home

    Name of at-home caregiver _____

☐ Attends adult day-care program

    ☐ Regular senior citizen day-care program

    ☐ Alzheimer's special care day-care program

☑ Living in assisted living residence

☐ Living in Alzheimer's special care unit of an assisted living residence

☐ Living in a long-term residential health care facility

☐ Living in Alzheimer's special care unit of a long-term residential health care facility

Medical diagnosis _Vascular Dementia, Type 2 Diabetes_

Cognitive/Memory assessment scores and/or dementia rating _MMSE-15_

Physical limitations _Profound Hearing Loss — frail with weak mobility_

Observation period _1-6-13 to 1-15-13_

Observation settings _Daily hourly observations in his residence_

Informant _Tom Burke_   Position _Social worker_

Section 2: Competency Levels

Record the level of current competencies by circling the number that best describes this individual's current level of interest and performance. This observation need not take place at one sitting but should be a record of a specific time period (for example, a 1-week period). If needed, use separate record forms to record an individual's performance in different locations (i.e., dining room, garden, shared meeting room, and during recreational, art, music, occupational, speech, and physical therapies). Use the Additional Notes section to note any changes in interest and engagement due to a specific activity, person, or environment.

Informants may choose to write descriptive notes of an individual's behavior and then record the written observations on the inventory. If the informant has not observed a specific activity, or questions an individual's ability to perform a specific task perhaps at another time or setting, the informant should record this in the column marked "Don't know" by circling the "?". Also, if a specific item does not apply due to the individual's physical limitations such as visual, motor, or hearing impairments, the informant should record this in the column marked "Not Applicable" by circling "NA."

At the end of each section of the inventory, the practitioner should total the number of points for that intelligence area and record the number in the Total Score box. Be sure to exclude the items in the "Not Applicable" and "Don't know" columns from this calculation. When the inventory is completed, write the total score of each intelligence area in the space provided in Section 3 of the inventory. Once these totals are recorded, circle the areas with the most points, then rank these in order in the spaces provided. The areas with the most points indicate the areas of greatest remaining competencies. Using this information, the practitioner can provide the individual with opportunities to use areas of preferences, remaining competencies, and possible potentials.

I. Verbal-Linguistic (Speaking, Reading, and Writing)

	Not Applicable	Never	Seldom	Frequently	Always	Don't know	
Speaking							
Participates in group discussions	NA	(0)	1	2	3	?	
Talks and reminisces with others	NA	0	(1)	2	3	?	Speaking Subscore:
Responds to verbal instructions	NA	0	(1)	2	3	?	
Uses polite expressions such as "Thank you," "Hello," "How are you?"	NA	0	1	2	(3)	?	**3**
Reading ★							
Reads books, newspapers, and other reading materials	NA	0	1	2	(3)	?	
Recognizes common signs such as *stop, go, no exit, exit, bathroom*	NA	0	1	2	(3)	?	Reading Subscore:
Responds to pictures and picture books by recognizing and naming pictures	NA	0	1	2	(3)	?	**9**
Writing							
Engages in writing activities such as maintaining a personal journal and writing letters and notes	NA	(0)	1	2	3	?	
Engages in written language activities such as completing crossword puzzles	NA	(0)	1	2	3	?	Writing Subscore:
Attempts to communicate by writing	NA	(0)	1	2	3	?	**0**

Total Score: **12**

(9 in reading)

Additional Notes:

Reading is a relative strength. Uses visual cues and printed signs and notes to understand oral commands. Has a daily routine of reading the newspaper!

II. Logical-Mathematical

	Not Applicable	Never	Seldom	Frequently	Always	Don't know
Responds to computers and electronic games	NA	(0)	1	2	3	?
Engages in board games such as checkers	NA	(0)	1	2	3	?
Engages in card games and other related activities such as dominoes	NA	(0)	1	2	3	?
Does simple math calculations such as counting items and keeping score	NA	0	1	2	(3)	?
Uses written lists and time schedules to prompt recall	NA	0	1	2	(3)	?
Performs best with order and reason	NA	0	1	2	(3)	?
Needs to know when daily events will occur	NA	0	1	2	(3)	?
Relies on step-by-step directions (oral or written)	NA	0	1	2	(3)	?
Engages in activities that involve puzzle completions and numbers	NA	(0)	1	2	3	?
Sorts objects by pattern, number, and shape	NA	(0)	1	2	3	?

Total Score: 15

Additional Notes:

Wants to know his schedule, but quickly forgets what he's told. Relies on written cues and a regular daily routine, esp. aware of when it's time to eat breakfast, lunch and dinner. Relies on his watch to check on the time and date. Still capable of doing mathematical calculations in his head, such as percentages and profits.

III. Visual-Spatial

	Not Applicable	Never	Seldom	Frequently	Always	Don't know
Visual Skill						
Notices interior decor and style and fashion (furniture, wall-hangings, colors, shapes, and clothes)	NA	0	1	(2)	3	?
Reads sentences, phrases, and words	NA	0	1	2	(3)	?
Responds to pictures and photographs	NA	0	1	2	(3)	?
Recognizes family photos	NA	0	1	(2)	3	?
Watches TV and videos	NA	0	1	2	(3)	?
Visual-Motor Skill						
Writes letters, sentences, phrases, or words	NA	(0)	1	2	3	?
Draws, doodles, paints, and colors	NA	(0)	1	2	3	?
Participates in most arts and crafts project	NA	(0)	1	2	3	?
Completes wooden puzzles	NA	(0)	1	2	3	?
Sorts objects in bins	NA	(0)	1	2	3	?

Total Score: **13**

Additional Notes:

Relies on written and visual cues. Aware of his surroundings and notices the dress and physical gestures & manners of people.

IV. Tactile-Kinesthetic

	Not Applicable	Never	Seldom	Frequently	Always	Don't know
Tactile						
Participates in arts and crafts projects (colors, traces, pastes, draws)	NA	(0)	1	2	3	?
Engages in activities such as cooking, baking, and sculpting	NA	(0)	1	2	3	?
Touches fabrics and textures and rummages through drawers	NA	(0)	1	2	3	?
Holds and fondles stuffed animals and dolls	NA	(0)	1	2	3	?
Kinesthetic						
Participates in exercise classes	NA	(0)	1	2	3	?
Uses exercise machines or equipment	NA	(0)	1	2	3	?
Engages in dance, sports, and walking activities	NA	(0)	1	2	3	?
Marches, sways, and moves head, arms, and feet to music	NA	(0)	1	2	3	?
Responds to massage therapy and occupational and physical therapies	NA	(0)	1	2	3	?
Paces and fidgets	NA	(0)	1	2	3	?

Total Score: *0*

Additional Notes:

Harris still is capable of walking with assistance.

Needs to be pushed in a wheelchair to get around the building.

Engaging and Communicating with People Who Have Dementia: Finding and Using Their Strengths, by Eileen Eisner. Copyright © 2013, by Health Professions Press, Inc.

V. Auditory-Musical

	Not Applicable	Never	Seldom	Frequently	Always	Don't know
Recites jingles, jokes, puns, rhymes, and poems	NA	0	(1)	2	3	?
Rhymes words; creates poems	NA	(0)	1	2	3	?
Plays a musical instrument or keeps time to music using musical instruments	NA	(0)	1	2	3	?
Responds to music therapy	NA	(0)	1	2	3	?
Sings songs; recalls words to songs	NA	(0)	1	2	3	?
Taps feet or claps hands to musical rhythms	NA	(0)	1	2	3	?
Responds to changes in a speaker's rone and pitch (i.e., shouting, whispering, high pitch)	NA	0	(1)	2	3	?
Listens to audiotapes and radio	NA	(0)	1	2	3	?
Soothed by soft music when agitated	NA	(0)	1	2	3	?
Reacts to loud noises	NA	(0)	1	2	3	?

Total Score: | 2 |

Additional Notes:

Profound hearing loss! Can barely participate in a conversation.
Needs to wear his hearing aids, but often forgets to put them on,
loses the aids or breaks the aids.

VI. Interpersonal

	Not Applicable	Never	Seldom	Frequently	Always	Don't know
Participates in group activities	NA	(0)	1	2	3	?
Responds to support groups	NA	(0)	1	2	3	?
Seeks company of others; doesn't like to sit alone; may ask, "Where's everybody?"	NA	(0)	1	2	3	?
Generally cooperates and shares	NA	0	(1)	2	3	?
Sympathetic to others' feelings	NA	(0)	1	2	3	?
Offers assistance to others (i.e., likes to give advice)	NA	(0)	1	2	3	?
Relaxes when in the company of others	NA	(0)	1	2	3	?
Needs to feel like part of a group	NA	(0)	1	2	3	?
Maintains polite social gestures and eye contact with others after losing ability to speak	NA	0	1	(2)	3	?
Appears to gain pleasure from watching others perform	NA	0	1	(2)	3	?

Total Score: 5

Additional Notes:

Doesn't socialize other than responding politely when greeted by others. He's a loner — eats alone at meals and never participates in group activities.

VII. Intrapersonal

	Not Applicable	Never	Seldom	Frequently	Always	Don't know
Responds to individual counseling	NA	(0)	1	2	3	?
Is intuitive or perceptive	NA	(0)	1	2	3	?
Works alone at own pace	NA	0	(1)	2	3	?
Produces creative and original work	NA	(0)	1	2	3	?
Expresses personal feelings	NA	0	1	(2)	3	?
Not concerned with what others think	NA	0	(1)	2	3	?
More responsive when talking about self	NA	0	(1)	2	3	?
Responds to verbal compliments	NA	0	(1)	2	3	?
Vulnerable self-worth and self-esteem	NA	(0)	1	2	3	?
Needs recognition and attention	NA	0	(1)	2	3	?

Total Score: 7

Additional Notes:

Needs to be approached in a respectful manner.

Always address him as "Mr. Rose," never call him "Harris"!

VIII. Naturalistic

	Not Applicable	Never	Seldom	Frequently	Always	Don't know
Cares for indoor plants	NA	(0)	1	2	3	?
Engages in outside gardening tasks	NA	(0)	1	2	3	?
Aware of weather and seasonal changes	NA	0	1	(2)	3	?
Responds to television shows and videos of natural scenery and animals (i.e., Discovery Channel)	NA	(0)	1	2	3	?
Responds to pictures of outdoor scenes, plants, flowers, and animals	NA	(0)	1	2	3	?
Appears to enjoy interacting with nature (i.e., watching birds on bird feeders)	NA	0	(1)	2	3	?
Responds to pet therapy and/or speaks to dogs, cats, or other pets	NA	(0)	1	2	3	?
Tends to sit outside (weather permitting) or in the solarium	NA	0	1	(2)	3	?
Responds and relaxes to audiotapes of nature sounds (i.e., rain, wind, waterfall, ocean waves)	NA	(0)	1	2	3	?
Seems less agitated when seated by a window; tends to look outside	NA	(0)	1	2	3	?

Total Score: ⟨ 5 ⟩

Additional Notes:

Seems to notice the weather. Definitely enjoys sitting or sleeping outside, weather permitting. Likes to sit in the sun!

Section 3: Summary of Competency Areas

Fill in the total score next to each intelligence. Circle the areas with the greatest number of points.

Verbal-Linguistic:	12	*(scored "9" in reading)*
Logical-Mathematical:	15	
Visual-Spatial:	13	
Tactile-Kinesthetic:	0	
Auditory-Musical:	2	
Interpersonal:	5	
Intrapersonal:	7	
Naturalistic:	5	

Areas of multiple intelligence with remaining competencies and preferences. Number 1 indicates the area of greatest remaining competency.

1. *Logical-Mathematical*
2. *Visual-Spatial (reading)*
3. *Verbal-Linguistic (reading)*
4. *Intrapersonal*

Caregiver Questionnaire and Checklist

▪▪

Section 1: Basic Information

Date: *1-6-13*   Individual's name: *Harris Rose*

Individual's preferred name or nickname: *Mr. Rose*

Informant's name and relation to individual: *Lena Jennings, daughter*

Section 2: Abilities and Interests

1. Please give a brief description of the individual's previous lifestyle (way of life):

   "Pillar of the community" — He was a successful businessman, community leader and philanthropist.

2. Please list the names of family members who are important to this individual. Include their relationship to the individual (i.e., Joe, brother):

   Lena, daughter   *Max, son-in-law*

   Martin, son   *Paula, granddaughter*

3. What was the individual's previous occupation(s)?

   Owned a successful auto dealership

4. List the individual's previous interests, talents, and hobbies:

   philantrophy

   sports — especially "The Yankees"

   avid reader of books, newspapers and magazines

5. Describe the individual's religious preferences:

   a. Is religion important to the individual? If so, what is the individual's religion?

   Yes, Catholic

   b. How did the individual participate in his or her religion? Did he or she attend services regularly or on occasion?

   Attended mass every Sunday

   c. Did the individual perform any special daily or weekly rituals?

   No

   d. Are religious holidays important to the individual? If so, which holidays in particular?

   Yes, Christmas

6. Did the individual have any pets? Does the individual like pets, such as cats, birds, or dogs?

   No

7. Does or did the individual play a musical instrument? If so, please describe.

   No

8. Does or did the individual enjoy singing and/or dancing? If so, please describe.

   No

9. Does the individual enjoy outdoors activities, such as gardening, walking, or sunbathing?

   Likes to sit and read outside when the weather is nice.

10. Does or did the individual have any special interest in sports, crafts, politics, current events, TV shows, theatre, and so forth. If so, what?

Likes to watch sports games, especially Yankee baseball games on TV.

11. Describe the individual's hearing. Does he or she wear a hearing aid? If so, is the hearing loss mild, moderate, or severe?

Severely hearing impaired — wears 2 hearing aids

12. Describe the individual's eyesight. Does he or she wear eyeglasses?

Needs to wear eyeglasses for all activities

13. Describe the individual's current motor skills.

    a. Is he or she mobile?

      Yes — but starting to have difficulty walking more than a few steps at a time

      a.i. If not, does he or she need a walker or wheelchair?

        Also, seems to have trouble with balance. Starting to use a wheelchair

    b. Can he or she button, zip, and snap clothes?

      Yes, but now with difficulty

    c. Can he or she use a pencil to write?

      Barely able to sign his name

    d. Can he or she use food utensils (a fork, etc.) properly?

      Yes

14. Describe the individual's current verbal skills.

    a. Can he or she still carry on a conversation?

       Very poorly! Only answers simple questions and keeps repeating the same questions.

    b. Is he or she bilingual? If so, what other language?

       No

    c. Does the individual use facial expressions and/or hand gestures to express him- or herself?

       Yes

    d. Does the individual's understanding improve or change when the speaker uses gestures? For example, if the speaker asks the individual if he or she wants a drink and the speaker pantomimes holding a glass and drinking.

       Yes

    e. Is the individual capable of expressing bodily needs, such as being thirsty or hungry or having to use the toilet.

       Yes

15. What is the best way to gain the individual's attention (e.g., a gentle touch, saying his or her name)?

    Call out his name and speak directly to his face. Look directly at him and speak in simple sentences. Use written notes to help him understand

16. Describe how the individual currently spends his or her day. Include any activities that seem to calm or relax the person.

    Has a daily schedule of washing, dressing, eating breakfast, watching TV, going to lunch, reading the newspaper, then watching TV until dinner time.

17. Please use this section to write any other information that you feel is important for staff to know about this individual.

Section 3: Lifespan Interests

Instructions: In the column labeled ACTIVITY, circle any activity that best describes the individual's current interests. Also, circle all of the Xs in the row to the right of the activity that you circle.

ACTIVITY	Verbal-Linguistic	Logical-Mathematical	Visual-Spatial	Tactile-Kinesthetic	Auditory-Musical	Interpersonal	Intrapersonal	Naturalistic
Animal care								X
Aromatherapy							X	X
Arts and crafts			X	X		X	X	
Baking			X	X				
Bird-watching			X					X
Board games	X	X	X			X		
Book club	X					X	X	
Carpentry		X	X	X				
Volunteer activities	X	X				X	X	
Child care						X	X	
Using a computer	X	X	X	X			X	
Cooking			X	X			X	
Creative Writing	X		X				X	
Crossword puzzles	X	X	X				X	
Current events	X					X	X	
Dancing				X	X	X	X	
Dinner parties	X					X		
Discussion groups	X					X		
Exercise classes				X				
Field trips				X		X		
Flower arranging			X	X				X
Folding laundry		X		X			X	
Gardening				X			X	X
Golf				X				X
Group bingo	X	X	X	X		X	X	
Indoor plant care								X
Interacting with children	(X)					(X)	(X)	
Journal writing	X		X				X	
Letter and note writing	X		X			X	X	
Listening to the radio	X				X			
Massages				X			X	
Meeting new people	X					X		
Mentoring others	X					X	X	
Listening to music					X			
Organizing drawers		X	X					
Painting, drawing, and coloring			X	X			X	

Section 3: Lifespan Interests *continued*

ACTIVITY	Verbal-Linguistic	Logical-Mathematical	Visual-Spatial	Tactile-Kinesthetic	Auditory-Musical	Interpersonal	Intrapersonal	Naturalistic
(Maintaining personal and family photo albums)			Ⓧ	Ⓧ			Ⓧ	
Working with plastic models		X	X	X				
Playing a musical instrument					X			
Psychotherapy	X						X	
Puzzles		X	X	X				
Reading books	X		X				X	
★ (Reading newspapers)	Ⓧ		Ⓧ				Ⓧ	
Relaxing to music					X			
(Religious rituals and ceremonies)	Ⓧ	Ⓧ	Ⓧ		Ⓧ	Ⓧ	Ⓧ	
Repairing household items		X	X					
Setting the table		X	X					
Sewing/knitting		X	X					
Shopping		X	X				X	
Singing	X				X	X	X	
Social functions	X					X		
Solitaire		X	X	X			X	
(Sports (playing or observing))		Ⓧ	Ⓧ	Ⓧ		Ⓧ		
(Sunbathing)							Ⓧ	Ⓧ
Swimming				X			X	X
Tennis			X	X				
Theater trips	X				X	X	X	
(Watching TV)	Ⓧ		Ⓧ		Ⓧ	Ⓧ	Ⓧ	
Yoga				X			X	X
TOTAL:	*4*	*2*	*5*	*2*	*2*	*4*	*6*	*1*

1. For each circled activity, total the number of circled Xs in the row to the right of the activity, and enter the count in the TOTAL row at the bottom of the table.

2. Fill in below the total score for each intelligence and circle the four intelligences with the highest number of points.

Verbal-Linguistic:	_4_		Auditory-Musical:	_2_
Logical-Mathematical:	_2_		Interpersonal:	_4_
Visual-Spatial:	_5_		Intrapersonal:	_6_
Tactile-Kinesthetic:	_2_		Naturalistic:	_1_

Engaging and Communicating with People Who Have Dementia: Finding and Using Their Strengths, by Eileen Eisner. Copyright © 2013, by Health Professions Press, Inc.

Section 3: Lifespan Interests *continued*

3. List below the four intelligences with the highest scores. The intelligence listed on line 1 indicates the area of greatest remaining interest for the individual.

a.i.1. *Intrapersonal* _____

a.i.2. *Visual-Spatial (reading)* _____

a.i.3. *Verbal-Linguistic (reading)* _____

a.i.4. *Interpersonal* _____

Personal Preferences Inventory

▪▪■▪▪■▪▪▪■▪▪■▪▪▪■▪▪■▪▪■▪▪▪■▪▪■▪▪▪■▪▪■▪▪■▪▪

Section 1: Basic Information

Date: *1-6-13*

Name: *Harris Rose*

Age: *95* Date of birth: *12-14-18*

Residence (home address or residential setting room number):
Gardens Assisted Living

Suite 218

Physical limitations such as wheelchair user, hearing impaired, visually impaired *Severe hearing loss;*
wears 2 hearing aids; limited mobility but can still walk; wears eyeglasses

Section 2: Personal Preferences

My favorite interests are
Reading the newspaper each day and watching TV

In the past I worked
I owned a successful business.

When I have free time I like to

Watch TV or take a nap

I have the most fun when

Children come to visit me.

I do not like the following activities:

I don't like group games or functions.

Section 3: Likes and Dislikes?

Instructions:

Each section describes a particular skill or interest. Read each statement. Then circle the number that best describes your feelings about this particular activity. Rate each activity on a scale from 0 to 3. **0 describes activities you do not like at all and 3 describes activities you really like to do.**

Some questions will pertain to your previous experiences; others will pertain to your current interests and talents. If you have never tried an activity and are unsure if you would enjoy it, circle the question mark in the "Don't know" column. At the end of each section, there is space for you to write any additional comments.

I. Verbal-Linguistic

	Strongly dislike	Do not like	Like	Like very much	Don't know
I participate in group discussions and/or book clubs.	(0)	1	2	3	?
I talk to other people.	0	(1)	2	3	?
I reminisce about when I was young.	0	1	(2)	3	?
I play word games such as Scrabble.	(0)	1	2	3	?
I listen. When you tell me something I usually respond.	(0)	1	2	3	?
I enjoy reading books, newspapers, and magazines.	0	1	2	(3)	?
I keep a personal family photo album.	0	1	(2)	3	?
I keep a personal diary or journal.	(0)	1	2	3	?
I write letters and notes.	(0)	1	2	3	?
I do crossword puzzles.	(0)	1	2	3	?

Total Score: *8*

Additional Notes:

_____

_____

_____

_____

_____

_____

II. Logical-Mathematical

	Strongly dislike	Do not like	Like	Like very much	Don't know
Electronic games and computer activities interest me.	(0)	1	2	3	?
I play card games and board games such as checkers.	(0)	1	2	3	?
Activities that involve finance such as investments, budgets, and maintaining accounting records interest me.	0	1	(2)	3	?
Gambling activities such as poker and horse racing interest me.	0	(1)	2	3	?
I follow a daily written schedule.	0	1	(2)	3	?
Being on time is important to me.	0	1	(2)	3	?
I use written lists to remind me of daily chores.	0	1	(2)	3	?
I always follow directions for activities such as cooking, crafts, and carpentry.	0	1	2	3	(?)
I complete jigsaw puzzles and build things.	(0)	1	2	3	?
I organize desk drawers and files.	0	(1)	2	3	?

Total Score: | 10 |

Additional Notes:

Likes "order" in his life

Needs a schedule of events

Time — is important to him

_____

_____

_____

III. Visual-Spatial

	Strongly dislike	Do not like	Like	Like very much	Don't know
I always notice room decor and furnishings.	0	(1)	2	3	?
I have a good sense of style and fashion.	0	(1)	2	3	?
I read books.	0	(1)	2	3	?
I keep a written journal and/or art portfolio.	(0)	1	2	3	?
I write notes and lists to help me remember items.	(0)	1	2	3	?
I usually remember what I see.	0	(1)	2	3	?
I look at pictures, graphics, and photo magazines as well as family pictures.	0	1	2	(3)	?
I work with my hands.	(0)	1	2	3	?
I doodle, draw, and paint.	(0)	1	2	3	?
I watch TV. My favorite shows are	0	1	2	(3)	?

Sports events, esp. baseball

Total Score: **10**

Additional Notes:

IV. Tactile-Kinesthetic

	Strongly dislike	Do not like	Like	Like very much	Don't know
I dance.	⓪	1	2	3	?
I walk or exercise daily.	⓪	1	2	3	?
I use exercise equipment.	⓪	1	2	3	?
When I hear music, I usually nod my head, tap my fingers, and move my feet.	⓪	1	2	3	?
I like to sew, bake, and cook.	⓪	1	2	3	?
I enjoy repairing and building things.	⓪	1	2	3	?
I like to get a massage.	⓪	1	2	3	?
I'm good at sports.	⓪	1	2	3	?
I touch fabrics and textures by doing such things as folding clothes and rummaging through drawers.	⓪	1	2	3	?
I walk around. Sitting in one place bores me.	⓪	1	2	3	?

Total Score: *0*

Additional Notes:

_____

_____

_____

_____

_____

_____

V. Auditory-Musical

	Strongly dislike	Do not like	Like	Like very much	Don't know
I play a musical instrument. If so, which instrument?	(0)	1	2	3	?
I sing.	(0)	1	2	3	?
I usually remember words to songs. Singing a tune helps me recall information.	(0)	1	2	3	?
I like jingles, jokes, puns, rhymes, and poems.	(0)	1	2	3	?
I usually remember what I hear.	(0)	1	2	3	?
Some music makes me want to dance.	(0)	1	2	3	?
I have a good ear for languages and recognizing foreign accents.	(0)	1	2	3	?
I like to listen to a cassette tape or the radio when I'm alone.	(0)	1	2	3	?
Soft music relaxes me.	(0)	1	2	3	?
Loud noises disturb my concentration.	0	1	(2)	3	?

Total Score: | 2 |

Additional Notes:

_____

_____

_____

_____

_____

VI. Interpersonal

	Strongly dislike	Do not like	Like	Like very much	Don't know
I participate in group discussions.	(0)	1	2	3	?
I like working with others.	(0)	1	2	3	?
I like participating in group activities.	(0)	1	2	3	?
I would rather sit with people than alone.	(0)	1	2	3	?
I usually cooperate and share with others.	0	(1)	2	3	?
I care about others' feelings.	(0)	1	2	3	?
I help others and give advice.	0	(1)	2	3	?
Friends are important to me.	(0)	1	2	3	?
In the past, I belonged to social clubs.	0	1	2	(3)	?
I enjoy watching others participate in musical or theatrical events.	0	1	(2)	3	?

Total Score: 7

Additional Notes:

Enjoys watching people, but does not like to participate in activities

Engaging and Communicating with People Who Have Dementia: Finding and Using Their Strengths, by Eileen Eisner. Copyright © 2013, by Health Professions Press, Inc.

VII. Intrapersonal

	Strongly dislike	Do not like	Like	Like very much	Don't know
I participate in counseling or psychotherapy.	(0)	1	2	3	?
I am intuitive.	(0)	1	2	3	?
I like to work alone and at my own pace.	0	1	(2)	3	?
I am creative.	0	(1)	2	3	?
I rely on my own judgment.	0	1	2	(3)	?
I enjoy being by myself. I relax better when I'm alone.	0	1	2	(3)	?
I don't care what others think of me.	0	1	2	(3)	?
I don't mind sharing my personal experiences with others.	0	(1)	2	3	?
I like when others compliment me.	0	1	(2)	3	?
I like recognition for my accomplishments.	0	1	2	(3)	?

Total Score: 18

Additional Notes:

Still has a strong sense of self. He's very independent and does not respond well when forced to do an activity. He is very resistant to particpate or move from is favorite recliner chair when he's tired or off his daily schedule.

VIII. Naturalistic

	Strongly dislike	Do not like	Like	Like very much	Don't know
I garden and care for indoor plants.	(0)	1	2	3	?
I always check weather reports. I sometimes plan my day by the weather.	(0)	1	2	3	?
I enjoy TV shows and videos of natural scenery and animals.	(0)	1	2	3	?
I look through picture books of outdoor scenes, plants, flowers, and animals.	0	(1)	2	3	?
I enjoy watching animals and birds in their natural habitats.	0	1	(2)	3	?
Animals are truly "man's best friends."	(0)	1	2	3	?
I talk to animals and sometimes plants.	(0)	1	2	3	?
I enjoy sitting in the sunlight.	0	1	2	(3)	?
I enjoy listening to audiotapes of nature sounds (i.e., rain, wind, waterfall, ocean waves).	(0)	1	2	3	?
When things get me down, a good nature walk makes me feel better.	(0)	1	2	3	?

Total Score: | 6 |

Additional Notes:

Likes to sit outside in the sun.

Engaging and Communicating with People Who Have Dementia: Finding and Using Their Strengths, by Eileen Eisner. Copyright © 2013, by Health Professions Press, Inc.

Section 4: Summary of Likes and Dislikes

Fill in the total score next to each intelligence area. Circle the areas with the greatest number of points.

Verbal-Linguistic: _____8_____

Logical-Mathematical: _____10_____

Visual-Spatial: _____10_____

Tactile-Kinesthetic: _____0_____

Auditory-Musical : _____2_____

Interpersonal: _____7_____

Intrapersonal: _____18_____

Naturalistic: _____6_____

This individual's interests and remaining potentials relate to the following intelligences, with Number 1 being the area with the greatest number of points:

1. _____*Intrapersonal*_____

2. _____*Logical–Mathematical*_____

3. _____*Visual–Spatial*_____

4. _____*Verbal–Linguistic*_____

Strength-Based Summary Sheet

Section 1: Basic Information

Name___Harris Rose_____ Date___1-15-13_____

Section 2: Summary Information

Intelligence	Informal Strength-Based Inventory Score	Caregiver Questionnaire and Checklist	Personal Preferences Inventory	Area of Strength (check top 4 areas with the greatest number of points)
Verbal-Linguistic	12	4	8	24
Logical-Mathematical	15	2	10	27
Visual-Spatial	13	5	10	28
Tactile-Kinesthetic	0	2	0	2
Auditory-Musical	2	2	2	6
Interpersonal	5	4	7	16
Intrapersonal	7	6	18	31
Naturalistic	5	1	6	12

Continued

Section 3:

_____ *Mr. Rose* _____ 's remaining competencies and current interests correlate with the following areas of multiple intelligence, with number 1 exhibiting the greatest potential:

1. *Intrapersonal*
2. *Visual-Spatial (reading)*
3. *Logical-Mathematical*
4. *Verbal-Linguistic (reading)*

Section 4:

According to the Caregiver Checklist, _____ *Mr. Rose* _____ still does or participates in the following activities:

1. *Reads newspapers*
2. *Enjoys religious services*
3. *Watches TV*
4. *Enjoys the company of children*

Dementia Care Staff Guide

> ### AVOID VERBAL DISAGREEMENTS!
> No one wins when you argue with someone who has memory problems. Change the subject or change the environment.

Patient's name _Harris Rose_   Room number _218_

Address the individual as _Mr. Rose or Mr. Harris_.

Circle phase of dementia: Mild

(Moderate)

Severe

To gain this individual's attention, use the following techniques

Call his name! Be sure to speak directly to him ("face to face").
Speak slowly and loudly.

This individual communicates by _speaking and using gestures_.

Remaining strengths _He has a strong independent spirit and relies on written signs and notes._

Create opportunities for the individual to use these strengths by doing the following: _Give him notes to remind him. Keep him on a rigid time schedule._

When the individual is agitated, use the following procedures to calm the individual:

1. _Use a firm, but gentle voice. Don't force him!_

2. _Walk away & tell him he has 5 more minutes. Come back every minute & say "now you have 4 more minutes" . . . and so on!_

The following interactions and activities should be avoided at all times:

1. _Never touch him when he's agitated_

2. _____

Memory Loss Caregiver Guide

▬▬▪▬▬▪▬▬▪▬▪▬▬▪▪▬▪▬▪▬▬▪▪▬▬▪▬▪▬▬▪▬▪▬▬▪▬▬▪▬▪▬▬▪

> **AVOID VERBAL DISAGREEMENTS!**
>
> No one wins when you argue with someone who has memory problems. Change the subject or change the environment.

_____Mr. Rose_____'s area of strength is *his strong sense of self and independent spirit*.

Use these strength-based activities daily:

1. *Use his awards and photos to help him reminisce*
2. *Give him a daily written schedule*
3. *Give him simple and direct instructions in writing*
4. *Give him the daily newspaper — discuss current events*
5. *Ask him for advice especially financial & business*

When _____*Mr. Rose*_____ gets agitated, use the following techniques to decrease any problem behaviors:

1. *Walk away & come back*
2. *Change the subject!*
3. *Give him a "count down," to an activity, i.e. "5 more minutes, 4 more*
4. *minutes, 3 more minutes . . . OK, now it's time to go! Tell him "why"*
5. *he needs to do something. Show him pictures to change the subject.*

Avoid the following *Direct confrontations!*
Don't yell!

Give your loved one opportunities to communicate by *Reading your written messages and responding to your questions*.

For immediate assistance and advice, call _____*Mrs. King*_____ at _____.
social worker

BARBARA S.

■■■■■■ ■■■■■■■ ■■■■■■■■ ■■■■■■ ■■■■■■

Age: 73

Medical diagnosis: Progressive Dementia

Phase of dementia: Mild to beginning moderate phase

Setting: Living at home with husband and with the aid of a daily professional caregiver and attending Adult Day Program

Assessment forms used:
Informal Geriatric Strength-Based Inventory, p. 56
Caregiver Questionnaire and Checklist, p. 66
Personal Preferences Inventory, p. 73

Guides used:
Memory Loss Caregiver Guide, p. 85

Note: The Dementia Care Staff Guide is not included because Barbara S. is currently living at home.

Informal Geriatric Strength-Based Inventory

▬▬▬▬ ▬ ▬▬▬ ▬ ▬▬ ▬ ▬▬ ▬ ▬▬ ▬ ▬▬ ▬ ▬▬ ▬ ▬▬ ▬ ▬▬ ▬ ▬▬ ▬ ▬▬ ▬ ▬▬ ▬ ▬▬ ▬ ▬

Section 1: Background Information

Individual's name _Barbara S._   Date _Jan. 10, 2013_

Date of birth _5/4/40_   Age _73_

Address or residential setting room number _5 Ashford Circle_

Naples, Florida

Check the appropriate boxes:

☑ Living at home

     Name of at-home caregiver _Husband, Jack, and private CNA, Hilda_

☐ Attends adult day-care program

     ☐ Regular senior citizen day-care program

     ☐ Alzheimer's special care day-care program

☐ Living in assisted living residence

☐ Living in Alzheimer's special care unit of an assisted living residence

☐ Living in a long-term residential health care facility

☐ Living in Alzheimer's special care unit of a long-term residential health care facility

Medical diagnosis _Alzheimer's Disease_

Cognitive/Memory assessment scores and/or dementia rating _mild to beginning moderate_

Physical limitations _none_

Observation period _1-3-13 to 1-10-13_

Observation settings _Adult Day Center and later at home with husband & aide_

Informant _Clara Smith_   Position _Recreational Therapist_

Section 2: Competency Levels

Record the level of current competencies by circling the number that best describes this individual's current level of interest and performance. This observation need not take place at one sitting but should be a record of a specific time period (for example, a 1-week period). If needed, use separate record forms to record an individual's performance in different locations (i.e., dining room, garden, shared meeting room, and during recreational, art, music, occupational, speech, and physical therapies). Use the Additional Notes section to note any changes in interest and engagement due to a specific activity, person, or environment.

Informants may choose to write descriptive notes of an individual's behavior and then record the written observations on the inventory. If the informant has not observed a specific activity, or questions an individual's ability to perform a specific task perhaps at another time or setting, the informant should record this in the column marked "Don't know" by circling the "?". Also, if a specific item does not apply due to the individual's physical limitations such as visual, motor, or hearing impairments, the informant should record this in the column marked "Not Applicable" by circling "NA."

At the end of each section of the inventory, the practitioner should total the number of points for that intelligence area and record the number in the Total Score box. Be sure to exclude the items in the "Not Applicable" and "Don't know" columns from this calculation. When the inventory is completed, write the total score of each intelligence area in the space provided in Section 3 of the inventory. Once these totals are recorded, circle the areas with the most points, then rank these in order in the spaces provided. The areas with the most points indicate the areas of greatest remaining competencies. Using this information, the practitioner can provide the individual with opportunities to use areas of preferences, remaining competencies, and possible potentials.

I. Verbal-Linguistic (Speaking, Reading, and Writing)

	Not Applicable	Never	Seldom	Frequently	Always	Don't know	
Speaking							
Participates in group discussions	NA	0	1	(2)	3	?	
Talks and reminisces with others	NA	0	1	2	(3)	?	**Speaking Subscore:**
Responds to verbal instructions	NA	0	1	2	(3)	?	
Uses polite expressions such as "Thank you," "Hello," "How are you?"	NA	0	1	2	(3)	?	*11*
Reading							
Reads books, newspapers, and other reading materials	NA	0	(1)	2	3	?	
Recognizes common signs such as *stop, go, no exit, exit, bathroom*	NA	0	1	2	(3)	?	**Reading Subscore:**
Responds to pictures and picture books by recognizing and naming pictures	NA	0	1	(2)	3	?	*6*
Writing							
Engages in writing activities such as maintaining a personal journal and writing letters and notes	NA	0	(1)	2	3	?	
Engages in written language activities such as completing crossword puzzles	NA	(0)	1	2	3	?	**Writing Subscore:**
Attempts to communicate by writing	NA	(0)	1	2	3	?	*1*

Total Score: *18*

Additional Notes:

_____

_____

_____

_____

_____

II. Logical-Mathematical

	Not Applicable	Never	Seldom	Frequently	Always	Don't know
Responds to computers and electronic games	NA	(0)	1	2	3	?
Engages in board games such as checkers	NA	(0)	1	2	3	?
Engages in card games and other related activities such as dominoes	NA	(0)	1	2	3	?
Does simple math calculations such as counting items and keeping score	NA	0	(1)	2	3	?
Uses written lists and time schedules to prompt recall	NA	0	(1)	2	3	?
Performs best with order and reason	NA	0	(1)	2	3	?
Needs to know when daily events will occur	NA	0	(1)	2	3	?
Relies on step-by-step directions (oral or written)	NA	0	1	(2)	3	?
Engages in activities that involve puzzle completions and numbers	NA	(0)	1	2	3	?
Sorts objects by pattern, number, and shape	NA	0	(1)	2	3	?

Total Score: ☐ 7

Additional Notes:

_____

_____

_____

_____

_____

III. Visual-Spatial

	Not Applicable	Never	Seldom	Frequently	Always	Don't know
Visual Skill						
Notices interior decor and style and fashion (furniture, wall-hangings, colors, shapes, and clothes)	NA	0	1	(2)	3	?
Reads sentences, phrases, and words	NA	0	1	(2)	3	?
Responds to pictures and photographs	NA	0	1	(2)	3	?
Recognizes family photos	NA	0	1	2	(3)	?
Watches TV and videos	NA	0	1	(2)	3	?
Visual-Motor Skill						
Writes letters, sentences, phrases, or words	NA	0	(1)	2	3	?
Draws, doodles, paints, and colors	NA	0	1	(2)	3	?
Participates in most arts and crafts project	NA	0	(1)	2	3	?
Completes wooden puzzles	NA	(0)	1	2	3	?
Sorts objects in bins	NA	(0)	1	2	3	?

Total Score: **15**

Additional Notes:

_____

_____

_____

_____

_____

IV. Tactile-Kinesthetic

	Not Applicable	Never	Seldom	Frequently	Always	Don't know
Tactile						
Participates in arts and crafts projects (colors, traces, pastes, draws)	NA	0	(1)	2	3	?
Engages in activities such as cooking, baking, and sculpting	NA	0	(1)	2	3	?
Touches fabrics and textures and rummages through drawers	NA	0	(1)	2	3	?
Holds and fondles stuffed animals and dolls	NA	(0)	1	2	3	?
Kinesthetic						
Participates in exercise classes	NA	(0)	1	2	3	?
Uses exercise machines or equipment	NA	(0)	1	2	3	?
Engages in dance, sports, and walking activities	NA	(0)	1	2	3	?
Marches, sways, and moves head, arms, and feet to music	NA	0	(1)	2	3	?
Responds to massage therapy and occupational and physical therapies	NA	0	(1)	2	3	?
Paces and fidget	NA	(0)	1	2	3	?

Total Score: 5

Additional Notes:

_____

_____

_____

_____

V. Auditory-Musical

	Not Applicable	Never	Seldom	Frequently	Always	Don't know
Recites jingles, jokes, puns, rhymes, and poems	NA	0	(1)	2	3	?
Rhymes words; creates poems	NA	0	(1)	2	3	?
Plays a musical instrument or keeps time to music using musical instruments	NA	0	1	2	(3)	?
Responds to music therapy	NA	0	1	2	(3)	?
Sings songs; recalls words to songs	NA	0	1	2	(3)	?
Taps feet or claps hands to musical rhythms	NA	0	1	2	(3)	?
Responds to changes in a speaker's tone and pitch (i.e., shouting, whispering, high pitch)	NA	0	1	2	(3)	?
Listens to audiotapes and radio	NA	0	1	(2)	3	?
Soothed by soft music when agitated	NA	0	1	2	(3)	?
Reacts to loud noises	NA	0	1	(2)	3	?

Total Score: **24**

Additional Notes:

*Loves to sing along with the radio or CDs, still plays piano —
still sings in her church choir.*

VI. Interpersonal

	Not Applicable	Never	Seldom	Frequently	Always	Don't know
Participates in group activities	NA	0	1	(2)	3	?
Responds to support groups	NA	0	1	(2)	3	?
Seeks company of others; doesn't like to sit alone; may ask, "Where's everybody?"	NA	0	1	2	(3)	?
Generally cooperates and shares	NA	0	1	2	(3)	?
Sympathetic to others' feelings	NA	0	1	(2)	3	?
Offers assistance to others (i.e., likes to give advice)	NA	0	1	(2)	3	?
Relaxes when in the company of others	NA	0	1	(2)	3	?
Needs to feel like part of a group	NA	0	1	2	(3)	?
Maintains polite social gestures and eye contact with others after losing ability to speak	NA	0	1	2	(3)	?
Appears to gain pleasure from watching others perform	NA	0	1	2	(3)	?

Total Score: ⟨25⟩

Additional Notes:

She's a people person!

VII. Intrapersonal

	Not Applicable	Never	Seldom	Frequently	Always	Don't know
Responds to individual counseling	NA	0	1	(2)	3	?
Is intuitive or perceptive	NA	0	1	(2)	3	?
Works alone at own pace	NA	0	(1)	2	3	?
Produces creative and original work	NA	0	(1)	2	3	?
Expresses personal feelings	NA	0	1	(2)	3	?
Not concerned with what others think	NA	0	(1)	2	3	?
More responsive when talking about self	NA	0	(1)	2	3	?
Responds to verbal compliments	NA	0	1	(2)	3	?
Vulnerable self-worth and self-esteem	NA	0	(1)	2	3	?
Needs recognition and attention	NA	0	1	(2)	3	?

Total Score: 15

Additional Notes:

_____

_____

_____

_____

_____

VIII. Naturalistic

	Not Applicable	Never	Seldom	Frequently	Always	Don't know
Cares for indoor plants	NA	0	1	(2)	3	?
Engages in outside gardening tasks	NA	0	(1)	2	3	?
Aware of weather and seasonal changes	NA	0	1	(2)	3	?
Responds to television shows and videos of natural scenery and animals (i.e., Discovery Channel)	NA	0	(1)	2	3	?
Responds to pictures of outdoor scenes, plants, flowers, and animals	NA	0	1	(2)	3	?
Appears to enjoy interacting with nature (i.e., watching birds on bird feeders)	NA	0	1	(2)	3	?
Responds to pet therapy and/or speaks to dogs, cats, or other pets	NA	0	1	(2)	3	?
Tends to sit outside (weather permitting) or in the solarium	NA	0	(1)	2	3	?
Responds and relaxes to audiotapes of nature sounds (i.e., rain, wind, waterfall, ocean waves)	NA	0	1	2	(3)	?
Seems less agitated when seated by a window; tends to look outside	NA	(0)	1	2	3	?

Total Score: 16

Additional Notes:

_____

_____

_____

_____

_____

Section 3: Summary of Competency Areas

Fill in the total score next to each intelligence. Circle the areas with the greatest number of points.

Verbal-Linguistic: _____*18*_____

Logical-Mathematical: _____*7*_____

Visual-Spatial: _____*15*_____

Tactile-Kinesthetic: _____*5*_____

Auditory-Musical: _____*24*_____

Interpersonal: _____*25*_____

Intrapersonal: _____*15*_____

Naturalistic: _____*16*_____

Areas of multiple intelligence with remaining competencies and preferences. Number 1 indicates the area of greatest remaining competency.

1. _____*Interpersonal*_____

2. _____*Auditory-Musical*_____

3. _____*Verbal-Linguistic*_____

4. _____*Naturalistic*_____

Caregiver Questionnaire and Checklist

■■

Section 1: Basic Information

Date: _1-8-13_____   Individual's name: _Barbara S._____

Individual's preferred name or nickname: _"Barb"_____

Informant's name and relation to individual: _Daughter, Jean_____

Section 2: Abilities and Interests

1. Please give a brief description of the individual's previous lifestyle (way of life):

   Wonderful homemaker, taught piano to children and sang in the church choir. Loves operas & muscial theatre.

2. Please list the names of family members who are important to this individual. Include their relationship to the individual (i.e., Joe, brother):

   Jack – Husband
   Jean – Daughter
   George – Son
   Linda – Sister & Bob, Brother-in-law

3. What was the individual's previous occupation(s)?

   Piano teacher, part-time at home residence

4. List the individual's previous interests, talents, and hobbies:

   Music – piano and choir. Enjoys listening to both classical & popular music. Loves "sing alongs."

Engaging and Communicating with People Who Have Dementia: Finding and Using Their Strengths, by Eileen Eisner. Copyright © 2013, by Health Professions Press, Inc.

5. Describe the individual's religious preferences:

   a. Is religion important to the individual? If so, what is the individual's religion?

   Loves singing hymns in church.

   b. How did the individual participate in his or her religion? Did he or she attend services regularly or on occasion?

   Attended services every Sunday — especially enjoyed being a choir member.

   c. Did the individual perform any special daily or weekly rituals?

   No.

   d. Are religious holidays important to the individual? If so, which holidays in particular?

   Loved Christmas and Easter family gathering and traditions.

6. Did the individual have any pets? Does the individual like pets, such as cats, birds, or dogs?

   No!

7. Does or did the individual play a musical instrument? If so, please describe.

   Played piano and was a piano teacher. Played piano at dance recitals, musical theatre productions and at all family parties.

8. Does or did the individual enjoy singing and/or dancing? If so, please describe.

   Music is very important to her. She loves to sing and listen to others sing.

9. Does the individual enjoy outdoors activities, such as gardening, walking, or sunbathing?

   not much

10. Does or did the individual have any special interest in sports, crafts, politics, current events, TV shows, theatre, and so forth. If so, what?

Loved muscial theatre — knows all the familiar show tunes.

11. Describe the individual's hearing. Does he or she wear a hearing aid? If so, is the hearing loss mild, moderate, or severe?

No

12. Describe the individual's eyesight. Does he or she wear eyeglasses?

No

13. Describe the individual's current motor skills.

   a. Is he or she mobile?

   Yes!

   a.i. If not, does he or she need a walker or wheelchair?

   No

   b. Can he or she button, zip, and snap clothes?

   Yes!

   c. Can he or she use a pencil to write?

   Yes!

   d. Can he or she use food utensils (a fork, etc.) properly?

   Yes!

14. Describe the individual's current verbal skills.

    a. Can he or she still carry on a conversation?

      yes, but limited!

    b. Is he or she bilingual? If so, what other language?

      speaks some French

    c. Does the individual use facial expressions and/or hand gestures to express him- or herself?

      very little

    d. Does the individual's understanding improve or change when the speaker uses gestures? For example, if the speaker asks the individual if he or she wants a drink and the speaker pantomimes holding a glass and drinking.

      She seems to understand more conversations & doesn't rely on gestures.

    e. Is the individual capable of expressing bodily needs, such as being thirsty or hungry or having to use the toilet.

      Yes!

15. What is the best way to gain the individual's attention (e.g., a gentle touch, saying his or her name)?

    Call her name!

16. Describe how the individual currently spends his or her day. Include any activities that seem to calm or relax the person.

    She likes to listen to the radio, play piano and watch old movies, esp. musicals.

17. Please use this section to write any other information that you feel is important for staff to know about this individual.

    She's a friendly woman, loving mother & wife. Music and family are very important to her.

Section 3: Lifespan Interests

Instructions: In the column labeled ACTIVITY, circle any activity that best describes the individual's current interests. Also, circle all of the Xs in the row to the right of the activity that you circle.

ACTIVITY	Verbal-Linguistic	Logical-Mathematical	Visual-Spatial	Tactile-Kinesthetic	Auditory-Musical	Interpersonal	Intrapersonal	Naturalistic
Animal care								X
Aromatherapy							X	X
Arts and crafts			X	X		X	X	
Baking			X	X				
Bird-watching			X					X
Board games	X	X	X			X		
Book club	X					X	X	
Carpentry		X	X	X				
Volunteer activities	X	X				X	X	
Child care						X	X	
Using a computer	X	X	X	X			X	
Cooking			X	X			X	
Creative Writing	X		X				X	
Crossword puzzles	X	X	X				X	
Current events	X					X	X	
Dancing				X	X	X	X	
Dinner parties	X					X		
Discussion groups	(X)					(X)		
Exercise classes				X				
Field trips				X		X		
Flower arranging			X	X				X
Folding laundry		X		X			X	
Gardening				X			X	X
Golf				X				X
Group bingo	X	X	X	X		X	X	
Indoor plant care								X
Interacting with children	(X)					(X)	(X)	
Journal writing	X		X				X	
Letter and note writing	X		X			X	X	
Listening to the radio	(X)				(X)			
Massages				X			X	
Meeting new people	(X)					(X)		
Mentoring others	X					X	X	
Listening to music					(X)			
Organizing drawers		X	X					
Painting, drawing, and coloring			X	X			X	

Section 3: Lifespan Interests *continued*

ACTIVITY	Verbal-Linguistic	Logical-Mathematical	Visual-Spatial	Tactile-Kinesthetic	Auditory-Musical	Interpersonal	Intrapersonal	Naturalistic
Maintaining personal and family photo albums			(X)	(X)			(X)	
Working with plastic models		X	X	X				
Playing a musical instrument					(X)			
Psychotherapy	X						X	
Puzzles		X	X	X				
Reading books	X		X				X	
Reading newspapers	X		X				X	
Relaxing to music					(X)			
Religious rituals and ceremonies	(X)	(X)	(X)		(X)	(X)	(X)	
Repairing household items		X	X					
Setting the table		X	X					
Sewing/knitting		X	X					
Shopping		X	X				X	
Singing	(X)				(X)	(X)	(X)	
Social functions	(X)					(X)		
Solitaire		X	X	X			X	
Sports (playing or observing)		X	X	X		X		
Sunbathing							X	X
Swimming				X			X	X
Tennis			X	X				
Theater trips	(X)				(X)	(X)	(X)	
Watching TV	(X)		(X)		(X)	(X)	(X)	
Yoga				X			X	X
TOTAL:	9	1	3	1	8	8	6	0

1. For each circled activity, total the number of circled Xs in the row to the right of the activity, and enter the count in the TOTAL row at the bottom of the table.

2. Fill in below the total score for each intelligence and circle the four intelligences with the highest number of points.

Verbal-Linguistic:	9	Auditory-Musical:	8
Logical-Mathematical:	1	Interpersonal:	8
Visual-Spatial:	3	Intrapersonal:	6
Tactile-Kinesthetic:	1	Naturalistic:	0

Section 3: Lifespan Interests *continued*

3. List below the four intelligences with the highest scores. The intelligence listed on line 1 indicates the area of greatest remaining interest for the individual.

a.i.1. *Verbal-Linguistic*

a.i.2. *Auditory-Musical*

a.i.3. *Interpersonal*

a.i.4. *Intrapersonal*

Engaging and Communicating with People Who Have Dementia: Finding and Using Their Strengths, by Eileen Eisner. Copyright © 2013, by Health Professions Press, Inc.

Personal Preferences Inventory

Section 1: Basic Information

Date: _Jan. 10, 2013_

Name: _Barbara S._

Age: _73_ Date of birth: _5-4-40_

Residence (home address or residential setting room number):

5 Ashford Circle

Naples, Florida

Physical limitations such as wheelchair user, hearing impaired, visually impaired _____ _No!_

Section 2: Personal Preferences

My favorite interests are

Family

Music, especially playing piano and singing.

In the past I worked

I taught piano to children in my home.

When I have free time I like to

Listen to music on the radio and CDs

play piano

watch people perform on stage, especially musicals

I have the most fun when

I'm playing piano or singing in a choir.

I do not like the following activities:

gardening

drawing

arts and crafts and cooking

Section 3: Likes and Dislikes?

Instructions:
Each section describes a particular skill or interest. Read each statement. Then circle the number that best describes your feelings about this particular activity. Rate each activity on a scale from 0 to 3. **0 describes activities you do not like at all and 3 describes activities you really like to do.**

Some questions will pertain to your previous experiences; others will pertain to your current interests and talents. If you have never tried an activity and are unsure if you would enjoy it, circle the question mark in the "Don't know" column. At the end of each section, there is space for you to write any additional comments.

I. Verbal-Linguistic

	Strongly dislike	Do not like	Like	Like very much	Don't know
I participate in group discussions and/or book clubs.	0	1	(2)	3	?
I talk to other people.	0	1	(2)	3	?
I reminisce about when I was young.	0	1	(2)	3	?
I play word games such as Scrabble.	0	(1)	2	3	?
I listen. When you tell me something I usually respond.	0	1	(2)	3	?
I enjoy reading books, newspapers, and magazines.	0	(1)	2	3	?
I keep a personal family photo album.	0	1	2	(3)	?
I keep a personal diary or journal.	0	(1)	2	3	?
I write letters and notes.	0	(1)	2	3	?
I do crossword puzzles.	(0)	1	2	3	?

Total Score: 15

Additional Notes:

_____

_____

_____

_____

_____

_____

II. Logical-Mathematical

	Strongly dislike	Do not like	Like	Like very much	Don't know
Electronic games and computer activities interest me.	(0)	1	2	3	?
I play card games and board games such as checkers.	(0)	1	2	3	?
Activities that involve finance such as investments, budgets, and maintaining accounting records interest me.	(0)	1	2	3	?
Gambling activities such as poker and horse racing interest me.	(0)	1	2	3	?
I follow a daily written schedule.	(0)	1	2	3	?
Being on time is important to me.	(0)	1	2	3	?
I use written lists to remind me of daily chores.	0	(1)	2	3	?
I always follow directions for activities such as cooking, crafts, and carpentry.	0	(1)	2	3	?
I complete jigsaw puzzles and build things.	(0)	1	2	3	?
I organize desk drawers and files.	(0)	1	2	3	?

Total Score: | 2 |

Additional Notes:

_____

_____

_____

_____

_____

_____

III. Visual-Spatial

	Strongly dislike	Do not like	Like	Like very much	Don't know
I always notice room decor and furnishings.	0	1	(2)	3	?
I have a good sense of style and fashion.	0	1	(2)	3	?
I read books.	0	(1)	2	3	?
I keep a written journal and/or art portfolio.	0	(1)	2	3	?
I write notes and lists to help me remember items.	0	(1)	2	3	?
I usually remember what I see.	0	(1)	2	3	?
I look at pictures, graphics, and photo magazines as well as family pictures.	0	1	(2)	3	?
I work with my hands.	0	(1)	2	3	?
I doodle, draw, and paint.	0	(1)	2	3	?
I watch TV. My favorite shows are	0	1	2	(3)	?

_____

_____

Total Score: | 15 |

Additional Notes:

_____

_____

_____

_____

_____

_____

IV. Tactile-Kinesthetic

	Strongly dislike	Do not like	Like	Like very much	Don't know
I dance.	0	1	②	3	?
I walk or exercise daily.	0	①	②	3	?
I use exercise equipment.	0	①	2	3	?
When I hear music, I usually nod my head, tap my fingers, and move my feet.	0	1	2	③	?
I like to sew, bake, and cook.	0	①	2	3	?
I enjoy repairing and building things.	0	①	2	3	?
I like to get a massage.	0	1	2	③	?
I'm good at sports.	⓪	1	2	3	?
I touch fabrics and textures by doing such things as folding clothes and rummaging through drawers.	⓪	1	2	3	?
I walk around. Sitting in one place bores me.	⓪	1	2	3	?

Total Score: | 12 |

Additional Notes:

_____

_____

_____

_____

_____

_____

V. Auditory-Musical

	Strongly dislike	Do not like	Like	Like very much	Don't know
I play a musical instrument. If so, which instrument?	0	1	2	(3)	?
I sing.	0	1	2	(3)	?
I usually remember words to songs. Singing a tune helps me recall information.	0	1	2	(3)	?
I like jingles, jokes, puns, rhymes, and poems.	0	1	(2)	3	?
I usually remember what I hear.	0	1	(2)	3	?
Some music makes me want to dance.	0	1	2	(3)	?
I have a good ear for languages and recognizing foreign accents.	0	1	(2)	3	?
I like to listen to a cassette tape or the radio when I'm alone.	0	1	2	(3)	?
Soft music relaxes me.	0	1	2	(3)	?
Loud noises disturb my concentration.	0	1	2	(3)	?

Total Score: | 27 |

Additional Notes:

_____

_____

_____

_____

_____

_____

VI. Interpersonal

	Strongly dislike	Do not like	Like	Like very much	Don't know
I participate in group discussions.	0	1	2	(3)	?
I like working with others.	0	1	2	(3)	?
I like participating in group activities.	0	1	2	(3)	?
I would rather sit with people than alone.	0	1	(2)	3	?
I usually cooperate and share with others.	0	1	(2)	3	?
I care about others' feelings.	0	1	(2)	3	?
I help others and give advice.	0	1	(2)	3	?
Friends are important to me.	0	1	2	(3)	?
In the past, I belonged to social clubs.	0	1	2	(3)	?
I enjoy watching others participate in musical or theatrical events.	0	1	2	(3)	?

Total Score: 26

Additional Notes:

VII. Intrapersonal

	Strongly dislike	Do not like	Like	Like very much	Don't know
I participate in counseling or psychotherapy.	0	(1)	2	3	?
I am intuitive.	0	1	(2)	3	?
I like to work alone and at my own pace.	0	(1)	2	3	?
I am creative.	0	1	(2)	3	?
I rely on my own judgment.	0	1	(2)	3	?
I enjoy being by myself. I relax better when I'm alone.	0	(1)	2	3	?
I don't care what others think of me.	(0)	1	2	3	?
I don't mind sharing my personal experiences with others.	0	1	(2)	3	?
I like when others compliment me.	0	1	(2)	3	?
I like recognition for my accomplishments.	0	1	(2)	3	?

Total Score: 15

Additional Notes:

_____

_____

_____

_____

_____

_____

VIII. Naturalistic

	Strongly dislike	Do not like	Like	Like very much	Don't know
I garden and care for indoor plants.	0	(1)	2	3	?
I always check weather reports. I sometimes plan my day by the weather.	0	(1)	2	3	?
I enjoy TV shows and videos of natural scenery and animals.	(0)	1	2	3	?
I look through picture books of outdoor scenes, plants, flowers, and animals.	(0)	1	2	3	?
I enjoy watching animals and birds in their natural habitats.	(0)	1	2	3	?
Animals are truly "man's best friends."	(0)	1	2	3	?
I talk to animals and sometimes plants.	(0)	1	2	3	?
I enjoy sitting in the sunlight.	0	1	(2)	3	?
I enjoy listening to audiotapes of nature sounds (i.e., rain, wind, waterfall, ocean waves).	0	1	2	(3)	?
When things get me down, a good nature walk makes me feel better.	0	(1)	2	3	?

Total Score: ☐ *8*

Additional Notes:

_____

_____

_____

_____

_____

_____

Section 4: Summary of Likes and Dislikes

Fill in the total score next to each intelligence area. Circle the areas with the greatest number of points.

Verbal-Linguistic:	*15*
Logical-Mathematical:	*2*
Visual-Spatial:	*15*
Tactile-Kinesthetic:	*12*
Auditory-Musical :	*27*
Interpersonal:	*26*
Intrapersonal:	*15*
Naturalistic:	*8*

This individual's interests and remaining potentials relate to the following intelligences, with Number 1 being the area with the greatest number of points:

1. *Auditory-Musical*
2. *Interpersonal*
3. *Verbal-Linguistic*
4. *Visual-Spatial*
5. *Intrapersonal*

Strength-Based Summary Sheet

Section 1: Basic Information

Name _Barbara S._   Date _1-8-13_

Section 2: Summary Information

Intelligence	Informal Strength-Based Inventory Score	Caregiver Questionnaire and Checklist	Personal Preferences Inventory	Area of Strength (check top 4 areas with the greatest number of points)
Verbal-Linguistic	18	9	15	42
Logical-Mathematical	7	1	2	10
Visual-Spatial	15	3	15	33
Tactile-Kinesthetic	5	1	12	18
Auditory-Musical	24	8	27	59
Interpersonal	25	8	26	59
Intrapersonal	15	6	15	36
Naturalistic	16	0	8	24

Continued

Section 3:

*Barbara*_____ 's remaining competencies and current interests correlate with the following areas of multiple intelligence, with number 1 exhibiting the greatest potential:

1. *Auditory-Musical*
2. *Interpersonal*
3. *Verbal-Linguistic*
4. *Intrapersonal*

Section 4:

According to the Caregiver Checklist, ___*Barbara*_____ still does or participates in the following activities:

1. *Plays Piano*
2. *Sings*
3. *Enjoys musical theatre and movies (musicals)*
4. *Listens to music CDs and radio*

Memory Loss Caregiver Guide

▀▄▀▄ ▀▄▀ ▄▀▄ ▀ ▄▀ ▄▀▄ ▀ ▄▀▄ ▀▄▀ ▄ ▄▀ ▄▀▄ ▀ ▄▀ ▄▀▄ ▀▄

AVOID VERBAL DISAGREEMENTS!

No one wins when you argue with someone who has memory problems. Change the subject or change the environment.

Barbara 's area of strength is _music and socializing_ .

Use these strength-based activities daily:

1. _Encourage her to play the piano._
2. _Provide her with social activities such as theatre._
3. _Provide her with opportunities for group singing._
4. _Provide her with opportunities to hear music and listen to both classical & show tunes._
5. _Encourage her to participate in group social activities._

When _Barbara_ gets agitated, use the following techniques to decrease any problem behaviors:

1. _Sing your instructions to her._
2. _Put on some soothing music CDs or radio program._
3. _Ask her to play the piano._
4. _Encourage her to join in a group activity or discussion._
5. _Show her photos of her family to change the subject._

Avoid the following _Yelling out instructions._
Don't leave her alone when she's upset.

Give your loved one opportunities to communicate by _giving her time to organize her thoughts into words._

For immediate assistance and advice, call _Clara Smith_ at _443-1782_ .
Recreation Therapist

STELLA P.

■ ■ ■■ ■ ■■ ■ ■■■ ■ ■■■ ■■ ■ ■■ ■ ■ ■ ■ ■■ ■■ ■ ■ ■ ■ ■ ■■ ■ ■■ ■ ■

Age: 75

Medical diagnosis: Alzheimer's disease

Phase of dementia: Mild phase (recently diagnosed)

Setting: Living at home with her son, daughter-in-law and two grandchildren

Assessment forms used: The SIMPLE

Note: Stella's son and daughter-in-law completed the SIMPLE to help them understand her current situation and plan activities that she could still enjoy. No other strength-based assessments have been used at this time.

The SIMPLE

(Simplified Inventory of Multiple Potential and Leisure Engagement)

▬▬▬▬▬▬▬▬▬▬▬▬▬▬▬▬▬▬▬▬▬▬▬▬▬▬▬▬▬

Section 1: Basic Information

Date: _2/14/13_ Individual's name: _Stella_

Individual's preferred name or nickname: _"Stel", Mom, Granny_

Informant's name and relation to individual: _Joe and Ellen Willis (son & daughter-in-law)_

Section 2: Current Competencies

Read each item carefully. Place a number 1 on the line to the right of each activity that this individual is currently interested in and is able to perform. Total the number of points in each group of activities (a–e) and place each total in the scoring section.

1. Verbal-Linguistic (speaking, reading, writing)

a. Likes to talk to others _1_

b. Participates in group discussions _1_

c. Enjoys reading _1_

d. Enjoys activities involving writing ____

e. Does word games, such as crossword puzzle _1_

Total: _4_

2. Logical-Mathematical (logic and reasoning)

a. Enjoys board games and cards _1_

b. Enjoys problem solving _1_

c. Excels in math calculations ____

d. Good with money management ____

e. Strong sense of time and time schedules ____

Total: _2_

3. Visual-Spatial (seeing and doing)

a. Very aware of design, décor, and dress _1_

b. Enjoys reading _1_

c. Enjoys writing ____

d. Enjoys drawing and other art activities ____

e. Enjoys watching t.v. and looking at photos _1_

Total: _3_

4. Tactile-Kinesthetic (body movement and sensation of touch)

a. Enjoys dancing ____

b. Enjoys exercising and walking ____

c. Enjoys doing tasks with hands
(building, sewing, fixing things) _1_

d. Enjoys sports ____

e. Doesn't like to sit for a long period of time ____

Total: _1_

Continued

Section 2: Current Competencies *Continued*

5. Auditory-Musical (listening involving pitch, tone, and rhythm)

a. Enjoys listening to music ___1___

b. Enjoys singing _____

c. Plays a musical instrument _____

d. Likes books on tape and listening to the radio ___1___

e. Speaks and/or recognizes other languages _____

Total: __2__

6. Interpersonal (social, likes people)

a. Enjoys being with people ___1___

b. Participates in group activities ___1___

c. Enjoys social events and parties ___1___

d. Enjoys being a part of a committee or group ___1___

e. Sensitive to the feelings of others ___1___

Total: __5__

7. Intrapersonal (self-knowledge, independence)

a. Likes to work alone _____

b. Has an independent personality ___1___

c. Likes to be a leader _____

d. Likes to talk about him- or herself _____

e. Needs to feel important _____

Total: __1__

8. Naturalistic (nature)

a. Enjoys being outdoors _____

b. Enjoys gardening _____

c. Enjoys caring for indoor plants ___1___

d. Loves animals ___1___

e. Responds to books and photos of nature _____

Total: __2__

Score

Place the totals from each of the 8 areas in the correct space below for that intelligence. Circle the areas with the greatest number of points.

Verbal-Linguistic: __4__

Logical-Mathematical: __2__

Visual-Spatial: __3__

Tactile-Kinesthetic: __1__

Auditory-Musical: __2__

Interpersonal: __5__

Intrapersonal: __1__

Naturalistic: __2__

List below the areas of multiple intelligence that currently rank the highest for this individual, starting with the highest score in the first space, followed by the next-lower scores in spaces 2, 3, and 4. Number 1 indicates this individual's greatest area of remaining interest and capability.

a.i.1. *Interpersonal (social)*

a.i.2. *Verbal-Linguistic (speaking & reading)*

a.i.3. *Visual-Spatial (seeing & doing)*

a.i.4. _____

Possible Ideas and Activities: Refer to Chapters 3, 4, and 5 of this book for specific recommendations.
Keep her involved with people!
1. Attend the Senior Center for daily senior lunch and other social events. 2. Participate in the Church Discussion groups, socials and luncheons. 3. Attend Knitting Club meetings every Tuesday at 3 pm. 4. Attend Monthly Book Club at the Library. 5. Play cards with family and friends. 6. Complete "easier" level crossword puzzles. 7. Buy an IPod and make a personalized play list of her favorite music.

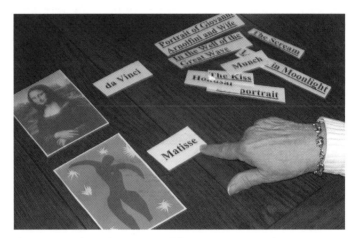

Playing a card matching game of famous painters and paintings
(visual-spatial/verbal-linguistic/intrapersonal strengths)

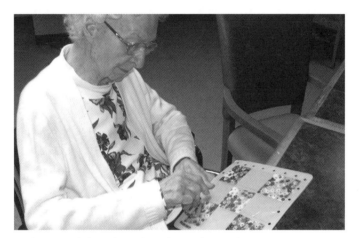

Quilting (tactile-kinesthetic/visual-spatial strengths)

Chapter 3
Strength-Based Interventions

▪▪▪▪▪▪▪▪▪▪▪▪▪▪▪▪▪▪▪▪▪▪▪▪▪▪▪▪▪▪▪▪▪▪▪

Practitioners, caregivers, and family members use strength-based interventions (SBI) to provide individuals with Alzheimer's disease opportunities for socialization and to successfully engage in meaningful conversations and activities throughout the progression of the disease. A rationale for all interactions is established by first identifying what an individual with Alzheimer's still can do and how to communicate with the person. In addition, an SBI approach enables family members and practitioners to diminish patient agitation and frustration by using techniques to draw upon and incorporate the individual's remaining strengths and abilities (multiple intelligence overview [the SIMPLE]), as well as his or her preferences and interests (Personal Preferences Inventory).

A strength-based framework enables practitioners to anticipate an individual's reaction to specific activities as well as to calm down a person when he or she is agitated, as shown in the following story of Dorothy:

Dorothy, an adult with Alzheimer's disease residing in a special care unit of a long-term health care facility, appeared agitated when presented with a group puzzle activity. She got out of her seat, throwing puzzle pieces and screaming unintelligible words. As the licensed practical nurse (LPN) redirected Dorothy to her seat, Dorothy's agitation increased. The speech–language pathologist (SLP), aware of Dorothy's verbal-linguistic preferences, intrapersonal strengths, and obvious cognitive and verbal limitations, intervened by speaking quietly and nodding in agreement to Dorothy's unintelligible screams. To redirect her, the SLP brought out Dorothy's personal memory book. Recognizing her personalized book of photographs, Dorothy stopped yelling but continued to utter incoherent words. The SLP interacted with Dorothy by smiling and nodding her head in agreement. Slowly, Dorothy was redirected to a quiet sitting area. She engaged in conversation with the SLP, pointing to her memory book of personal photographs and uttering words such as "kid," "baby," and "mom." The LPN, witnessing this interaction, asked the SLP, "How did you calm down Dorothy?" The SLP replied, "Even though her ability to talk is limited, Dorothy still wants to speak. She needs to relate to people. She seems less agitated when others appear to understand her feelings. She needs recognition. When left unattended and faced with difficult tasks she becomes frightened and agitated. Puzzle completions are too challenging for her. Screaming is the only means Dorothy has to express her frustration. A gentle word along with a sympathetic gesture (nod of the head) enables Dorothy to connect with another person. Using these strategies, along with a personal memory book, will diminish Dorothy's agitation."

Dorothy not only still prefers verbal-linguistic activities but also exhibits a remaining strength in intrapersonal intelligence. Using a strength-based intervention to keep individuals such as Dorothy participating in life's experiences is the essence of the intervention itself.

The goal of all activity planning is intervention, not simply occupying time. Practitioners must ask and answer the question, "Why is this person doing this activity?" Intervention implies that there is a rationale for every activity at any given time. A strength-based intervention answers the question of why the person is doing an activity by providing practitioners and family members with a rationale for planning appropriate leisure activities for the person and when possible prompting pleasant conversations. If the answer to the question is vague, then the appropriateness of the activity is suspect. For example, if the Informal Geriatric Strength-Based Inventory indicates that an individual has no tactile-kinesthetic aptitude or interests, it does not mean that he or she should automatically be eliminated from all dancing experiences. For a person who still retains interpersonal and musical capabilities, the experience of observing others dance and listening to music is beneficial. The musical and social experience becomes a meaningful activity for the passive observer as well as the active dancer. The answer to why the individual is involved in dance therapy is that he or she enjoys the social, interpersonal experience of watching others perform as well as the personal experience of listening to music. Even though the individual's participation is limited to that of an observer, he or she is engaged in a personally meaningful experience.

Providing Appropriate Strength-Based Interventions Throughout the Progression of Dementia

As mentioned in Chapter 1, people who have a neurodegenerative disease experience three distinct phases: mild, moderate, and severe. Successful strength-based activities match a person's preferences with his or her diminishing cognitive functioning and capabilities. Once practitioners, family members, and caregivers are familiar with an individual's interests and current competencies, they can provide activities in a reverse developmental progression. As Jolene Brackey states, "As the disease progresses, a person with Alzheimer's gets younger and younger and younger in his mind." (2007, p. 18) For example, a patient with tactile-kinesthetic preferences who is unable to perform traditional arts and crafts activities may be encouraged to mold clay or to handle squeeze balls. These basic tactile-kinesthetic experiences would offer the individual, who may be in the severe phase, a stimulating activity with few cognitive demands.

Understanding a person's preferences and waning competencies enables practitioners, family members, and caregivers to plan activities that promote success. The following sections describe how to match an individual's remaining preference with his or her diminishing skills.

Verbal-Linguistic Preferences

Individuals who still exhibit verbal-linguistic intelligence frequently demonstrate a preference for verbal and written language tasks and may benefit from a variety of activities throughout the progression of Alzheimer's. During the mild phase of the disease, these individuals take part in activities such as writing journal entries, an autobiography, or poetry, participating in group discussions, and reading. During the moderate phase of the disease, they can benefit from creating a personal memory book of photographs as well writing corresponding descriptive sentences. During the moderate phase, these individuals may enjoy reading books of high interest to them that are at low reading level (e.g., books written for high school students with learning disabilities). Individuals in the severe phase who still possess verbal-linguistic preferences may benefit from looking at personal memory book photographs to recall long-term memories of loved ones and family events.

> Esther, in the severe phase of dementia, attempted to communicate by laughing, smiling, pointing, and uttering sounds. She did not use words spontaneously. Her family members began to doubt that she still recognized them. When presented with a memory book of personal photographs, however, Esther exhibited some remaining verbal-linguistic function by pointing to some of the photos and spontaneously saying single words. Once, while sitting with her son, Esther pointed to a photograph of him and said, "You." The single word "you" reassured Esther's son that his mother still knew him.

Providing Esther with a verbal-linguistic prompt such as the memory book enabled her to engage in a brief but extremely meaningful interaction with her son.

Logical-Mathematical Preferences ▮▮▮▮▮▮▮▮▮▮▮▮▮▮

Individuals who still possess logical-mathematical preferences typically re-spond to activities that involve order and schedules. During the mild phase of a neurodegenerative disease, these individuals respond to board games, com-puter activities, card games, jigsaw puzzles, and organizational tasks, such as filing and maintaining daily schedules. Those in the moderate stage of the disease participate in activities such as tic-tac-toe, bingo, jumbo dominoes, and simple jigsaw puzzles. Individuals in the late stage respond to memory books of family photographs, picture lotto, bingo games, and large wooden puzzles as well as to sorting and classifying objects.

Visual-Spatial Preferences ▮▮▮▮▮▮▮▮▮▮▮▮▮▮▮▮

Those who still have visual-spatial intelligence and preferences react to visual cues. Individuals in the mild phase of Alzheimer's can participate in games such as concentration and bingo as well as painting, drawing, playing computer games, and engaging in crafts activities. Those in the moderate phase enjoy engaging in games such as picture dominoes and charades as well as painting, coloring, tracing, and drawing activities. Individuals in the severe phase of the disease can participate in Velcro tic-tac-toe, jumbo toss, and bingo games in addition to activities that involve coloring books, finger-painting, molding clay, and play dough.

Tactile-Kinesthetic Preferences ▮▮▮▮▮▮▮▮▮▮▮▮

Individuals with a neurodegenerative disease who exhibit remaining tactile-kinesthetic preferences respond to physical movement and touch. Those in the mild phase engage in dance, exercise classes, and creative dramatic ac-tivities in addition to sports, such as bowling, golf, and tennis, as well as the Nintendo Wii computer games (Wii Fit, Wii Sports). During the mild phase, individuals participate in crafts activities, such as building airplane models and molding and sculpting activities. Those in the moderate phase respond to games such as beanbag toss, Velcro tic-tac-toe, darts, and card-matching as well as other activities ranging from sorting and folding laundry to creating personal memory boxes. Patients in the severe phase of Alzheimer's respond to baby dolls and plush toys that are specifically designed for adults with cog-nitive loss as well as activities that involve touching boards, discovery boxes, large wooden puzzles, Velcro horseshoes, beanbags, squeeze balls, textures, and fabrics.

Auditory-Musical Preferences ▨▨▨▨▨▨▨▨▨▨▨▨▨▨

People with Alzheimer's who still possess auditory-musical intelligence and preferences are sensitive to sounds, music, and languages. Those in the mild phase enjoy playing games such as Name That Tune, playing musical instruments, and participating in sing-alongs. These individuals also enjoy dance and music therapies, exercising, walking, and relaxing to music, and listening to radio shows and audiobooks. Those in the moderate phase of the disease participate in a variety of activities that involve music, including participating in sing-alongs, playing musical toy instruments, and listening to music on an audiotape or CD or to stories with an accompanying picture book. Patients in the severe phase of the disease may respond to looking at a personal memory book while listening to an audiotape that describes each photograph. They also typically respond to plush animals and baby dolls that have sound effects. Music can usually ease agitation in those who still possess auditory-musical intelligence during the final phase of the disease.

Interpersonal Preferences ▨▨▨▨▨▨▨▨▨▨▨▨▨▨

Adults who have a neurodegenerative disease and who still exhibit interpersonal intelligence and preferences benefit from being in, and feel best when in, the company of others. They typically respond positively to social activities, such as discussions, creative drama, book clubs, and storytelling. Those in mild stage participate in group games, such as Life, Clue, Outburst, What's My Line?, and bingo. They also engage in art projects, such as making gifts for loved ones or creating collages of personally meaningful pictures. Individuals in the moderate phase participate in group discussions, group trips, role-playing activities, and most social activities. Those in the more severe stage of dementia still need to socialize and interact with others. These older adults respond to intergenerational and pet therapies, and may also respond to holding and caressing baby dolls and plush toys.

Intrapersonal Preferences ▨▨▨▨▨▨▨▨▨▨▨▨▨▨

Those with Alzheimer's who exhibit intrapersonal intelligence prefer independent, self-paced activities. Individuals in the mild phase engage in independent activities such as writing daily journal or diary entries and completing independent art projects. They may also enjoy writing an autobiography, maintaining a sketchbook, making a family tree, keeping a personal calendar, and creating a collage of personal items. Individuals with moderate dementia may prefer playing card games, such as solitaire. They may also enjoy engaging in independent verbal or written sentence completions, such as "When I was young _____."; "I'm the happiest when I _____."; and "My children _____." Those in the late stage perform best when engaged in personalized tasks, such as looking through a memory book or wallet of family photographs or a memory box of personal mementos. Viewing family home videos might also prompt recall.

Naturalistic Preferences

Individuals who possess naturalistic preferences respond to activities that involve nature. During the mild phase of Alzheimer's, individuals respond to outdoor activities such as picnics, nature walks, and gardening. These individuals also enjoy books and projects that involve nature, science, and animals. Individuals in the moderate phase enjoy television shows about nature and animals, such as programs on the Discovery Channel and Animal Planet. These individuals benefit from pet therapy as well as other animal and pet care activities, such as maintaining an aquarium or ant farm. They also benefit from picture and coloring books about science, animals, and nature, as well as lotto, dominoes, and bingo games that include animal and nature pictures. Individuals with severe dementia can enjoy walking (if possible), sitting, and touching items in an outside courtyard or inside solarium, as well as sitting by a bay window to view the outdoors. They can participate in puzzle and card-matching activities that involve animals and nature. Viewing DVDs or photos of nature and animals as well as listening to audiotapes or CDs of nature sounds (e.g., wind, rain, ocean waves) can ease agitation for an individual with remaining naturalistic preferences.

Individualized Strength-Based Activities

This section organizes a wide array of leisure activities according to a strength-based model, and can be used to assist family members and caregivers in selecting appropriate activities and materials that the individual still can do and enjoys. Activities are grouped according to each of the eight intelligences and are then organized in a reverse developmental order (from higher- to middle- to lower-level functioning), which allows the practitioner, caregiver, or family members to select appropriate and meaningful activities for an adult with waning cognitive abilities throughout the progression of the dementia. This section also includes both individual and group activities. The following information may be used as a guide to facilitate and simplify the task of personalizing activities to meet the needs of each individual. In addition, once family members and caregivers have administered and scored the SIMPLE, they can use the information in this section to complete the "Ideas and Possible Activities" portion of the SIMPLE.

Verbal-Linguistic (Speaking, Reading, Writing) ▨▨▨

Higher Level

Word Game Activities ▨

- Play games (20 Questions, Outburst or Outburst Jr., Scrabble or Scrabble Jr., Sentence Scrabble, Clue, word-matching lotto, reminiscence bingo, magnet poems)

Individual Writing Activities ▨

- Email friends and family
- Solve crossword puzzles and other word puzzles
- Write personal biography
- Write in a journal
- Participate in creative writing, storytelling, and story writing
- Write letters to pen pals and family members
- Write puns, limericks, and jokes
- Send text messages via a cell phone

Verbal Language Activities ▨

- Participate in group discussions about current events, the daily newspaper, and idioms and expressions
- Participate in informal debates and brainstorming sessions
- Discuss nostalgic topics
- Join a book club
- Participate in a comedy club (listen to and tell jokes)
- Serve as the recording secretary in a club meeting
- Play games that promote verbal discussion, such as Trivial Pursuit

Group and Art Activities ▨

- Compile a book of creative writings and poetry
- Compile an anthology of jokes, puns, and limericks

- Develop pen pal relationships with other residents or schoolchildren
- Write letters of interest to important figures or companies
- Write seasonal plays and newsletters
- Write a weekly or monthly column for the local newspaper, senior citizen paper, or healthcare facility newsletter

Middle Level

Individual Word Game Activities ▨

- Play games such as Boggle Jr., Sentence Scrabble, Scrabble Jr., Blurt Jr., and Clue Jr.

Individual Writing Activities ▨

- Complete fill-in-the-blank poems or a personal journal or diary (sentence or paragraph completions)
- With assistance, create a scrapbook of personal photographs and hand-written comments
- Unscramble sentences of familiar expressions or famous quotes
- Complete a personal book titled "Grandmother Remembers" (or "Grand-father Remembers")
- Reminisce about nostalgic topics by matching a photograph of a famous individual or event to a descriptive sentence or well-known quotation
- Match a cartoon drawing to a written joke

Group Discussion Activities ▨

- Use physical props as discussion topics (e.g., old record player, telephone, radio)
- Read and discuss well-known book classics based on the age of the individual
- View and discuss old classic films
- Participate in choral readings

Group Activities ▨

- Compose a group story for which each participant adds to the story. A discussion leader gives written copies of the story to each participant, and the participants take turns reading the story to the group.

- Compile a collection of completed poems or simple creative stories (e.g., "My Favorite Holiday")
- Write stories using colorful magazine pictures as prompts
- Display creative writings on a bulletin board
- Write and share life stories

Lower Level

Game and Toy Activities ▨

- Hold, touch, and discuss plush animals that have sound effects
- Play color, shape, or picture lotto games
- Play Outburst Jr., Boggle Jr., Sentence Scrabble
- Solve beginner word searches

Individual Activities (may require assistance) ▨

- Read books written for children ages 7 to 12 (choose mature topics or well-known poems or stories)
- Read magazines and books with large pictures and titles
- Complete journal, poem, and sentence fragments, such as "I like my _____", "I seem to be _____", or "Sometimes I like to _____."
- With direct assistance, create a memory book of personal photographs and write short sentences or single descriptive words for each photograph
- Create scrapbook collections of magazine pictures that can be used as conversation starters

Group Discussion Activities ▨

- Reminisce about nostalgic topics, such as old movies, sports heroes, musicians, etc.
- Use large posters as conversation starters
- Use photographs and physical props as discussion topics (e.g., World War II army uniform, bridal veil, wedding photographs)
- View and discuss old movies
- Use books and magazines with large photographs for discussion topics

Group and Art Activities ▨

- Create picture collages

- Create picture menus from magazine pictures and photographs

- Listen to storytellers

- Listen to recordings of old radio shows or watch DVDs of old television shows (e.g., *You Bet Your Life!*, *Burns and Allen*, *I Love Lucy*, *Father Knows Best*)

Logical-Mathematical (Logic, Reasoning) ▨▨▨▨

Higher Level

Game Activities ▨

- Play board games, such as checkers, chess, and backgammon

- Play card games, such as poker, solitaire, bingo, lotto

- Play computer games and dominoes

Individual Activities ▨

- Create a library by organizing books and using a sign-in for visitors

- Make a family tree

- Write daily journal or diary entries

- Organize personal information in a notebook or daily or hourly time schedule

- Compute simple mathematical story problems

- Organize and work at a desk or work center (e.g., simple filing, use a calculator, use a computer)

- Play sports with soft sponge balls and dart games with Velcro targets

- Complete puzzles, tangrams, Sudoko, logic games

Group and Art Activities ▨

- Act as timekeeper or scorekeeper for group games

- Complete paint-by-numbers projects

- Play mathematical games

- Create graphs and maps

- Construct plastic models

- Complete carpentry projects

Middle Level

Game Activities ▨

- Play large-size checkers, jumbo bingo, or lotto (road signs, geography, money, addition, subtraction, multiplication, and division lotto), jumbo dominoes, Chutes and Ladders, large-size Chinese checkers, games with money (Monopoly or Monopoly Jr.)

Individual Activities ▨

- Play number-matching card games and card games that involve sorting and classifying pictures, objects, colors, shapes, coins, etc.

- Complete maze and dot-to-dot paper and pencil activities

- Build with jumbo LEGOs

- Place stickers on large calendars to label daily schedules

- Organize events using picture cards and personal organizers

- Play basic-level computer games

Group and Art Activities ▨

- Participate as the group scorekeeper, using a calculator to tally scores

- Complete picture pattern cards

- Work on parquetry and puzzles

- Sort, count, and organize arts and crafts supply bins

- Sort and classify objects by size, shape, and color

- Do dot-to-dot pencil and paper activities

- Use wooden craft sticks to make objects

- Construct simple plastic models

Lower Level

Game Activities ▨

- Play primary-level lotto games (e.g., survival road signs, colors, shapes, alphabet, numbers, money), Candy Land, Chutes and Ladders, jumbo checkers, jumbo bingo (picture card, number, shape, money, and color bingo), and Velcro dart games (act as scorekeeper for the games)

Individual Activities ▦

- Build with jumbo LEGOs

- Match color cubes to picture pattern cards

- Classify objects and picture cards according to function, shape, or color

- Create memory books and memory wallets to share with others

- Create personal organizer and daily personalized pictorial calendar (see Appendix D, Attainment Company)

- Create large picture menus and calendars as visual cues in the dining room

- Use manipulatives for sensory stimulation and to sort, classify, and organize objects into bins

- Organize desk drawers, magazine racks, and files

Group and Art Activities ▦

- Complete simple, primary-level wooden puzzles

- Use wooden eye–hand tracking materials

- Sort objects by color, size, shape, and number using plastic sorting trays or sorting boxes

Visual-Spatial (Seeing, Doing) ▦▦▦▦▦▦▦▦▦

Higher Level

Game Activities ▦

- Play board games, such as Pictionary; Win, Lose, or Draw; Concentration; and Guess Who?

- Play dominoes, bingo, charades, jacks, and darts

Individual Activities ▦

- Complete peg board activities

- Play computer games (see Chapter 5 for detailed suggestions)

- Participate in computer keyboarding, typewriter, and Morse code activities

- Complete jigsaw puzzles

- Draw with an Etch-a-Sketch, Magna Doodle, or View-Master Super Sketch Projector

Paper, Pencil, and Paint Activities ▨

- Complete mazes, pictures, cartoons, paint-by-number sets, diagrams, and map drawings
- Make a family tree
- Draw a map of his or her room or a shared communal room
- Create a montage of pictures depicting his or her life story
- Assist in creating seasonal bulletin board displays
- View CDs and/or family home videos to recall significant family events and individuals

Group Discussion Activities ▨

- Use picture cues as conversation starters
- Participate in listen-and-draw activities
- Use picture and written organizers to recall daily schedules and events

Art Activities ▨

- Create personal collages
- Draw, paint, and color
- Sculpt clay
- Complete basic knitting, sewing, and quilting activities
- Construct plastic models of planes, boats, and cars
- Make paper flowers
- Create and use memory boxes and memory books

Middle Level

Game Activities ▨

- Play Chutes and Ladders, Candy Land, dominoes, picture dominoes, tic-tac-toe, charades, large-size number bingo, Velcro jumbo darts, and Guess Who?

Individual Activities ▨

- Complete jumbo peg board designs with matching cards
- Create miniature dollhouses
- Complete easy pencil and paper exercises, such as mazes and dot-to-dot activities

- Solve jumbo puzzles

- Sequence stories and picture cards

- Use an Etch-A-Sketch or Magna Doodle

- Sort greeting cards according to holiday or personal event (birthday, anniversary, etc.)

- Sort picture cards according to topic, color, and shape

- Clip discount coupons from newspapers and sort them by category

- Alphabetize and organize files and rolodex cards

- Organize library books by category

- Write descriptive sentences under each photo in a personal memory book

Groups Discussion Activities ■■

- Use large nostalgic posters and familiar objects as conversation starters

Art Activities ■■

- Paint, color, trace, and draw

- Sculpt and model clay

- Color jumbo picture posters

- Knit and sew

- Organize and sort yarn by color and sort fabrics by texture

- Create fabric and picture collages

Lower Level

Game Activities ■■

- Play Velcro tic-tac-toe; jumbo toss game (with beanbags and a large board); jumbo Candy Land; picture, color, and shape jumbo bingo and dominoes

Individual Activities ■■

- Use Mood Wall (Touch Me) (see Flaghouse in Appendix D)

- Complete aerial tabletop mazes

- Sort pictures, shaped and colored tiles, wooden puzzles, and stacking boxes

- Use jumbo wooden peg boards

- Use matching, sorting, and counting games

- Use jumbo magnetic paper doll sets and Color Form activities

- Complete felt board activities

- Use sequence-and-picture association cards

- Use a variety of visual products, such as classic lava lamps, chalkboard and chalk, large picture books, and kaleidoscopes

- Use picture placemats designating utensil placement to set the table

- Use memory books

- Watch family videos

- Use an audio card reader

Group Discussion Activities ▨

- Use bright, bold, simple, and nostalgic posters and familiar objects to prompt discussion

- Use videos of familiar activities or old movies to relax and prompt recall

- Use environmental wall cues in the form of attractive, simple, and theme-related posters to designate and recall the functions of specific rooms

Art Activities ▨

- Complete jumbo coloring books and children's watercolor books

- Use play dough and molding clay

- Complete finger-painting activities

- Participate in pencil and paper tracing activities, preschool mazes, and dot-to-dot activities

- Make photo and magazine picture collages

- Make fabric collages

- Complete felt board activities

- Use Velcro activity boards and string beads

Tactile-Kinesthetic (Body Movement, Sensation of Touch) ▬▬▬▬▬▬▬▬▬▬▬▬▬▬▬

Higher Level

Individual Activities ▨

- Participate in physical, occupational, massage, and aromatherapy therapies

- Manage own personal grooming, such as bathing, washing, combing or brushing hair, brushing teeth, shaving, and putting on makeup

- Help with laundry and housecleaning tasks, such as putting clothes in the washer or dryer, folding clean clothes, putting clothes away, cleaning and polishing shoes and furniture, vacuuming, and dusting

- Participate in activities using exercise equipment

- Walk, arrange flowers, cook, and bake

- Create miniature dollhouses

- Decorate a room for seasonal events and holidays

- Construct with LEGOs

- Care for an ant farm

Group Games and Activities

- Play Simon Says, Hokey Pokey, musical chairs, charades, and Follow the Leader

- Participate in a puppetry performance

- Participate in physical exercises and sports, such as tennis, volleyball, badminton, bowling, golf, and dancing

- Participate in gardening activities

- Participate in creative dramatics

Group Discussion Activities

- Express ideas through body movement, facial expressions, and hand gestures

- Talk while participating in physical activities, such as group walks and trips

- Speak while cooking, painting, sculpting, and engaging in craft activities

- Try on costumes and act out dramatic roles

- Sit in a comfortable lounge chair with pillows

Art Activities

- Try origami as well as cutting, carving, molding, sculpting, and pasting activities

- Build model airplanes

- Weave baskets

- Create sand art
- Distribute and collect art supplies during recreational arts and crafts

Middle Level

Individual Activities ▓▓

- Sort and fold clothes
- Create a memory box of personal items
- Organize and sort miniatures and other objects using sorting trays and bowls
- Use an abacus
- Use manipulation boards; shape towers

Game Activities ▓▓

- Play Concept Town (see PRO-ED in Appendix D), Clue Jr., Chutes and Ladders, beanbag activities, Velcro beanbag target game, Velcro tic-tac-toe, and tactile touch and play lotto games
- Play with sponge rackets, indoor sports bats and balls, and wooden peg boards with matching cards
- Play Velcro sports and dart games, and beach ball volley game with Velcro paddles and balls

Group Discussion Activities ▓▓

- Use physical cues, such as gentle taps, to focus attention on group discussion
- Act out ideas
- Touch objects of various textures and shapes while speaking
- Use physical prompts to promote conversations
- Pantomine
- Use Bubble Maker: Floating Bubbles (see Flaghouse in Appendix D)

Lower Level

Game and Object Activities ▓▓

- Manipulate squeeze balls, discovery boxes, and baby dolls and plush toys designed for adults

- Play with large wooden puzzles, ring toss games, horseshoes, Velcro bean-bag games, and soft toss sets, such as children's bowling

Individual Activities ■■

- Use a vibrating pillow, small handheld plastic fan, large wooden puzzles, fuzzy tactile puzzles, and pom-pom balls in rubber and fleece
- Use Bubble Maker: Floating Bubbles
- Use giant and small rain sticks

Individual Pastimes Activities ■■

- Participate in aromatherapy and massage therapies
- Rummage through drawers, touching various objects and fabrics
- Make a memory box of personally significant objects, such as house and car keys, library card, wallet, etc., of varying sizes and textures to serve as a conversation starters
- Sit in a glider or rocking chair
- Use physical way-finding environmental cues (while walking to a room or common areas)

Art Activities ■■

- Make a collage of varied textured fabrics
- Finger paint and complete water-coloring activities and sponge art
- Manipulate play dough or clay; squeeze balls
- Touch textured materials and fuzzy stickers

Auditory-Musical (Listening that involves pitch, tone, and rhythm) ■■■■■■■■■■■■■

Higher Level

Game Activities ■■

- Play Name That Tune and Name That Holiday (naming the seasonal song), the telephone game, and finger and action rhymes
- Participate in sing-alongs and listening games using a tape recorder
- Play musical instruments

Individual Activities ▨

- Participate in individual and group music therapy

- Listen to music while writing, drawing, dressing, eating, and walking

- Use a headset to listen to music tapes of CDs while exercising, strolling, and relaxing

- Listen to nostalgic music to prompt recall of relevant personal events

- Participate in activities that involve rhymes and poems

Group and Art Activities ▨

- Participate in music and dance therapies

- Participate in line dances, such as the Electric Slide, High Hat Joe, and the Hokey Pokey, as well as ethnic dances, such as the Hora, Tarantella, etc.

- Listen to background music while working on art projects

- Participate in a singing group or choir

Middle Level

Game Activities ▨

- Play Name That Tune and Hear and See (use audiocassettes of familiar sounds from different environments with matching pictures (see Flaghouse in Appendix D)

- Participate in karaoke (stereo-assisted sing-alongs)

Individual Activities ▨

- Enjoy a private listening center composed of audiotapes, CDs, and headsets to listen privately to audiobooks and music

- Use musical instruments, giant rain sticks, small xylophones, tabletop chimes, music boxes, and hanging chimes

- Use a memory book of personalized photographs as well as a coordinated audiotape or CD to describe each photograph

- Listen to audio messages created by family members when feeling lonely and stressed

Group Discussion and Art Activities ▨

- Use wireless microphone set with speakers to prompt attention and recall

- Complete multiple-choice activities, matching the picture of the speaker to the correct audio presentation

- Use props with sound effects (i.e., coughing ashtray) to enhance discussions

- View DVDs of popular musicals

- Use exaggerated vocal pitch and volume to encourage participation in group activities

- Complete fill-in-the-blank activities, such as completing rhymes, chants, axioms, familiar expressions, and poems

Lower Level

Game Activities ■■

- Play the xylophone, bells, and other musical instruments

- Move body, clap hands, and tap fingers to music

Individual Activities ■■

- Use talking and moving plush animals designed especially for adults with cognitive impairments

- Use shaking toys to produce sounds, such as jingle balls, rattles, and bells

- Attend to visitors after hearing a doorbell

- Listen to audiotape of favorite music, life story, family messages, or coordinated description of a memory book

- Use simple books for elementary school children with bold pictures as well as poetry and rhyme books with accompanying audiotapes, such as *Brown Bear, Brown Bear: What Do You See?*

Group and Art Activities ■■

- View videos of historical speeches and events to prompt recall for group discussions

- Use pictures of well-known or popular singers as multiple-choice activity to select the individual who is singing a particular song

- Participate in "listen and draw" exercises using familiar poems and rhymes

- Use wireless microphone set with speakers to prompt attention

- Use props with sound effects (e.g., animal sounds, sirens) to enhance group discussions

- View videos of old musicals

- Listen to music to ease agitation

Interpersonal (Social) ▨▨▨▨▨▨▨▨▨▨▨▨▨▨▨

Higher Level

Game Activities ▨

- Play board games, such as Scruples, Life, Clue, 20 Questions, and Outburst, and play dominoes and Velcro darts

Individual Activities ▨

- Participate in an early-stage Alzheimer's support group

- Participate in a senior citizen, religious, or spiritual group

- Help others residing in a long-term care facility

- Interact with children, such as reading

- Write in a journal daily

Group Discussion and Art Activities ▨

- Participate in group therapy, storytelling, dramatics, and role-playing activities

- Join a daily discussion group

- Work under supervision on community-related project, such as helping the homeless

- Participate in group trips and picnics

- Make a group photograph collage of all friends, family, or residents of long-term care facility

- Make a group quilt or participate in a similar group activity

- Collaborate with others on a group art project

- Help others decorate a shared communal room

- Volunteer for community service with assistance from a college student, caregiver, or family member

Middle Level

Games ▨

- Play Outburst Jr., Clue Jr., bingo, tic-tac-toe, dominoes, Velcro darts, 20 Questions, Simon Says, Hokey Pokey, Follow the Leader, and card games
- Participate in a puppetry performance or role-playing and creative dramatics

Individual Activities ▨

- Greet visitors
- Create a photo album of group activities
- Assist others in decorating a facility for seasonal holidays
- Participate in a pet therapy and intergenerational program
- Participate in daily writing exercises in the form of sentence completions

Group and Art Activities ▨

- Participate in social activities, such as choral and dance activities
- Participate in all appropriate group activities, such as joining a choir, collaborating on a group mural, and planting a group garden
- With assistance, work on scrapbooking activities
- View family photographs and home videos and share them with others

Lower Level

Game Activities ▨

- Play picture lotto, picture matching, picture bingo, picture dominoes, Simon Says, Hokey Pokey, Follow the Leader, and jumbo tic-tac-toe

Individual Activities ▨

- Participate in pet therapy (if the individual previously enjoyed domestic pets)
- Hold and touch baby dolls and plush toys designed specifically for adults with cognitive impairments
- Use a home life center that includes a baby carriage, crib, dressing table, and supplies
- Sit with others in a shared communal room

- Use a personal memory book or memory wallet of photographs to prompt recall

- Communicate with others by using gestures and eye contact

- Attempt simple wooden puzzles that depict people

- Use animated plush toys and hand puppets designed specifically for adults with cognitive impairments to start conversations

Group and Art Activities

- Participate in group intergenerational activities and puppetry, musical, and dramatic performances

- Sing with a group

- Participate in group outings, dinners, and special events

- Greet visitors

- Make collages of magazine photographs showing groups of people

Intrapersonal Intelligence (Self-knowledge, Independent Spirit)

Higher Level

Games

- Play Concentration, Go Fish, Monopoly, solitaire, checkers, chess, Clue, bingo, 20 Questions, dominoes, and Jeopardy

Individual Activities

- Maintain a daily journal

- Write an autobiography

- Write an opinion book (e.g., What I Think)

- Write letters, notes, and emails to family members and friends

- Write and use a personal calendar of daily and weekly activities

- Maintain financial journals

- Write personal anecdotes next to meaningful photographs in a memory book

- Create a collage of personal papers and photographs to decorate a personal living space

- Write creative poetry
- Complete crossword puzzles, word finds, mazes, puzzles, drawings, and wood carvings
- Create a plastic model
- Knit, sew, and cook
- Read books

Group Discussion Activities ▨

- Participate in group discussions by sharing personal opinions and feelings about past events
- Participate in conversations about values, beliefs, and behaviors
- Offer advice and opinions
- Participate in group psychotherapy
- Share personal reminiscences and experiences

Art Activities ▨

- Draw, paint, and collect items that are personally meaningful
- Create products that enable expression of inner feelings
- Use room displays that depict personal experiences and achievements (e.g., personal photographs, awards)

Middle Level

Games ▨

- Play Concentration, Go Fish, Old Maid, Monopoly Jr., solitaire, checkers, Clue Jr., 20 Questions, Outburst Jr., jumbo dominoes, word and picture dominoes, bingo, and Jeopardy

Individual Activities ▨

- Write in a personal journal or diary with a fill-in-the-blank format
- Write memoirs using a sentence-completion format
- Use a simplified fill-in-the-blank personal calendar as a reminder of daily activities
- Create and read a memory book of photographs and written descriptions
- Create a personal picture collage

- Decorate a personal living space with meaningful memoirs

- Compose simple poetry

- Participate in any independent activity that can be done successfully, such as simple crossword puzzles, drawing, tracing, painting, sculpting, gardening, wood carving, constructing models, knitting, sewing, cooking, puzzles, and reading books

Lower Level

Game Activities

- Play picture lotto, picture bingo, and picture dominoes

- Complete wooden puzzles

Individual Activities

- Participate in pet therapy and psychological counseling

- Look through a personal memory book of photographs

- Look through a box of personal mementos and objects to prompt recall

- Watch personal family videos of previously meaningful family events

Group and Art Activities

- Participate in group events and discussions by discussing personal feelings and beliefs

- Offer individual verbal compliments

- Recall previous experiences by listening to stories from caregivers

- Assist individuals in expressing feelings

- Create opportunities for individuals to feel important

- Participate in group intergenerational activities

Naturalistic (Nature)

Higher Level

Games and Activities

- Participate in a wide array of outdoor activities, such as picnics, nature walks, field trips, and gardening

- Care for indoor plants, domestic pets, terrarium, fish bowls, and ant farms

- Participate in pet therapy activities
- Participate in science activities that involve plants and nature
- Participate in gardening activities
- Build plastic models of the human body, plants, and animals
- Sort and organize books and pictures of animals and plants
- Read books, journals, and magazines about nature, animals, and plants
- Watch videos and listen to audiotapes of nature scenes and sounds
- Watch television shows about animals

Group Discussion Activities ▨

- Play group question and answer games that include science and nature topics
- Participate in discussions that involve nature-related topics, such as animals, ecology, meteorology, and geography

Middle Level

Games and Activities ▨

- Participate in outdoor activities, such as picnics, nature walks, and field trips
- Participate in gardening exercises, such as seeding, raking, mowing, picking flowers, etc.
- Care for houseplants and flowers
- Participate in pet therapy
- Play animal and plant picture games, such as lotto, dominoes, and bingo
- Sort animal and plant pictures
- Use adult coloring books that include pictures of animal and plant life
- Read illustrated books on science, botany, and biology
- Complete jigsaw puzzles of plants and animals
- Sculpt animals and plants
- Collect and organize a picture scrapbook of plants, animals, and nature scenes

- Watch DVDs and listen to CDs of nature scenes and sounds, such as the sound of rain, a waterfall, or trees blowing in the wind

- Watch animal- and nature-related television shows and movies

Lower Level

Games and Activities

- Under supervision, participate in outside activities

- Walk and sit in an outside setting, such as a courtyard or patio

- Participate in appropriate gardening chores, such as simple digging and planting activities

- Under direct supervision, mow the lawn using a manual lawn mower

- Gather fallen leaves, sweep the path or sidewalk, and pick flowers

- Sit by a bay window to observe weather and seasonal changes

- Hold animal plush toys

- Decorate with silk plants and flowers when no longer capable of caring for live plants

- Look through large picture books on nature, plants, and animals

- Participate in arts and crafts activities that involve coloring, painting, and sculpting figures of animals and plants

- Create poster collages of animal and plant pictures

- Complete simple wooden puzzles of animals and plants

- Complete picture-sorting activities that involve animals and plants

- Match pictures using animals and plant lotto, dominoes, and bingo games

- Watch videos and listen to audiotapes of nature scenes and sounds, such as the sound of rain, a waterfall, or trees blowing in the wind

- Watch animal- and nature-related television shows and movies

Individualizing Group Strength-Based Activities

Leisure and recreational activities for people with Alzheimer's and other dementias may be grouped according to a specific multiple intelligence as well as to a combination of intelligences. Strength-based intervention enables practitioners to modify programs according to the interests and capabilities of all individuals. Planning appropriate activities for groups of people involves coordinating activities to match a combination of intelligences. Some activities may provide for all eight areas of intelligence, while others might involve only one or two areas. For example, using a personalized photo album accommodates all eight intelligences, while dancing caters to the auditory-musical, tactile-kinesthetic, and interpersonal areas of intelligence.

The goal of group activity is to engage each participant in a meaningful and successful experience. When activities are planned according to an individual's current capabilities and preferences, he or she is more apt to participate. A strength-based model enables practitioners to select the appropriate activity for each group member. Strength-based activities encourage individuals in a group to engage in a positive social experience by succeeding through their own multiple-intelligence strength.

Practitioners may choose to implement a theme-based approach to recreational, communication, dance, activity, and music therapy. By organizing programs into thematic units, practitioners can offer individuals with Alzheimer's an array of multisensory activities to reinforce a specific topic or theme. The goal of a theme unit is to keep participants in touch with reality. For example, holiday themes assist individuals in recalling holidays and events. Professionals may reinforce a Fourth of July holiday theme with dance and music activities such as patriotic sing-alongs and marches. Group discussion topics, enhanced by visual and physical prompts such as posters, pictures, American flags, picture books, and patriotic videos, coordinate with the Fourth of July theme. Activity therapy reinforces the patriotic Fourth of July theme with activities such as creating American flags from fabrics or paper and coloring red, white, and blue American flags. A Fourth of July picnic with coordinated decorations, music, and entertainment provides all group members with opportunities to reminisce.

Other popular themes are movies, famous celebrities and sports figures, occupations, travel, families, children, music, sports, foods, traditions, animals, nostalgia art (e.g., Norman Rockwell illustrations), original television shows (*Lassie, Father Knows Best, The Honeymooners, Cars*), and vintage jewelry, objects, and styles.

This section provides samples of seasonal theme-related, strength-based group activities that practitioners can assist an individual with Alzheimer's in doing. Bear in mind that this is only a sampling. Also, specific seasonal activities are only appropriate in geographic locations where seasonal changes occur. In areas where there are few seasonal changes, practitioners may organize theme units by holidays and regional events.

Fall

Verbal-Linguistic Activities

- Participate in outside group discussions on fall memories that include conversation starters such as "In fall, I like to . . . " and "Every autumn, I see . . . " as prompts for creative writing and poetry activities.

Logical-Mathematical Activities

- Participate in outdoor experiences that involve collecting, sorting, counting, classifying, and charting plants, trees, animals, and birds.

- Create a fall scrapbook of pressed leaves or flowers organized and labeled according to type of tree or flower.

Visual-Spatial Activities

- Create leaf collages, draw what the person sees outdoors, and participate in leaf rubbings and printing activities as well as flower arranging and pressing activities.

Auditory-Musical Activities

- Listen and sing songs related to the fall season.

- Play musical instruments in the outside environment.

- Use sticks, leaves, and small gardening tools as musical instruments.

- Make musical rattles and shakers from dried seeds and beans in various sealed cups and containers.

Tactile-Kinesthetic Activities

- Rake leaves, mow the lawn, weed, pick vegetables from a garden, pick apples, and plant small shrubs along a designated outside wandering path.

- Engage in arts and crafts activities, such as making birdhouses, leaf rubbings, and potpourri out of dried flowers and spices as well as arranging dried flowers and pressing flowers.

Interpersonal Activities

- Engage in group activities, such as walking, planting, and gardening.

- Participate in fall picnics and social events, such as apple picking.

- Participate in all group discussions as well as group arts and crafts activities.

Intrapersonal Activities

- Contribute to group discussions by sharing personal opinions, ideas, and memories.

- Plant individual flower patch or pick flowers for the person's room. An individual with remaining intrapersonal preferences typically responds to activities that are personally meaningful. Practitioners might encourage these individuals to participate by using verbal prompts such as "Let's make potpourri for your room. The potpourri will make your room smell beautiful."

Naturalistic Activities

- Engage in all outdoor activity, including group walks, short trips, and picnics.

- Participate in planting, gardening, and bird-watching activities.

- Use natural media, such as leaves, seeds, herbs, and flowers, for arts and crafts activities.

- Create leaf rubbings, make potpourri out of dried flowers and spices, press flowers, and arrange dried flowers.

Depending on the facility's geographic location, therapists may expand the fall activities by providing the group with a fall apple picking experience. These outdoor experiences may be expanded into a group activity of baking an apple pie, which involves a wide array of multiple intelligences, such as the following:

- Picking apples: tactile-kinesthetic, naturalistic, interpersonal, and intrapersonal

- Sorting apples: logical-mathematical, visual-spatial, tactile-kinesthetic, and naturalistic

- Washing and drying apples: tactile-kinesthetic

- Cutting apples and making apple filling (reading recipes): tactile-kinesthetic, verbal-linguistic, logical-mathematical, visual-spatial, interpersonal, and intrapersonal

- Making pie dough: tactile-kinesthetic, verbal-linguistic, logical-mathematical, visual-spatial, interpersonal, and intrapersonal

• Smelling the pie baking and eating the pie: enjoyed by all individuals

To expand the fall theme, take photos of outings and create a bulletin board display of these shared experiences. Label each photograph with the person's name and a description of the activity. Use the display board as a memory prompt to encourage individuals to talk about their experiences and to recall the current season. At the end of the fall season, place all photographs and written descriptions into a group memory book, which will serve as a group discussion starter to prompt recall as well as a visual reminder of shared experiences.

Winter

In a geographic location where there is no winter season, practitioners can incorporate the traditional Christmas, Chanukah, Kwanzaa, and Three Kings Day holidays into a group theme unit. The purpose of a theme-related unit of activities is to increase an individual's awareness of time and events. Using a seasonal theme also enables individuals to interact socially, recall previous winter seasons, and to focus on what is currently taking place. Of course, practitioners provide groups with appropriate and meaningful themes based on the culture of a particular facility.

Verbal-Linguistic Activities

• Participate in group reading and discussion activities based on winter themes, such as winter sports, previous winter blizzards, winter holidays, and so on.

• Write and send greeting cards for the holiday season.

Logical-Mathematical Activities

• Maintain a weather calendar to chart the temperature and weather conditions.

• Keep a schedule of winter events and social activities.

• Count and sort seasonal decorations that would be of interest to the person.

Visual-Spatial Activities

• Participate in all seasonal arts and crafts.

• Create a snowman and snowflake mobile from various tactile materials.

• Decorate a bulletin board with seasonal decorations that would be of interest to the person.

Tactile-Kinesthetic Activities

- Decorate for the seasonal holiday and create and wrap seasonal presents.

- Bake traditional holiday treats.

- Participate in costume activities, such as trying on or organizing various winter coats, jackets, scarves, gloves, and hats.

- When and where appropriate, build a snowman in an enclosed patio area.

Auditory-Musical Activities

- Sing and play seasonal songs and other music.

- Participate in sing-alongs.

- Play a "name that winter song" game.

Interpersonal Activities

- Take part in group discussions that encourage recall of winter memories.

- Use seasonal posters, books, and classic holiday movies to stimulate conversations and recall.

Intrapersonal Activities

- Participate in group discussions that stimulate the sharing of perceptions and recall of winter recollections.

- Create a collage of personal photographs that show past winter experiences.

Naturalistic Activities

- Create a floral or plant arrangement for the winter season.

- When weather and personal stamina permit, participate in outdoor activities such as shoveling snow or building a snowman in an enclosed patio area.

- Maintain a bird feeder by the person's bedroom window.

To elaborate on the winter or holiday theme, photograph all seasonal-related activities and events and create a winter holiday bulletin board display of these shared experiences. Label each photograph with the person's name and a description of the activity. Use the display board as a memory prompt to encourage individuals to talk about their experiences and to recall the current season. At the end of the season, add the photographs to a group memory book, which will serve as a group discussion starter to prompt recall as well as a constant reminder of shared group experiences.

Spring

In most geographic regions the spring season is a celebration of rebirth and life. It is time to plant, observe the trees and flowers budding, commence outdoor activities, spring clean, and celebrate Easter, Passover, and Mother's Day.

Verbal-Linguistic Activities

- Weather permitting, participate in outdoor group discussions.

- Use pictures, photographs, and other visuals as well as hands-on gardening activities to stimulate conversations.

- Discuss or write about spring sayings and topics such as the following:

  The early bird catches the worm.
  Birds of a feather flock together.
  April showers bring May flowers.
  It's raining cats and dogs.
  Spring fever

Logical-Mathematical Activities

- Design and plan a garden. Compute the amount of time, money, and yard space necessary for this activity.

- Maintain a weekly calendar of gardening chores.

- If capable, for individuals in the severe phase of Alzheimer's, count, sort, and organize seeds according to size and shape, or categorize individual seed packets according to flowers, herbs, and vegetables.

Visual-Spatial Activities

- Engage in group discussions using visual prompts such as drawings, photographs, videos, and pictures books on spring events. Large reproductions of well-known artwork (Vincent van Gogh's *Sunflowers*) would encourage reminiscences about spring.

- Participate in arts and crafts activities, such as coloring books of flowers, plants, or trees.

- Create and paint a bird feeder.

- Make tissue paper flowers, fabric butterflies, and macramé plant hangers.

Tactile-Kinesthetic Activities

- Assist in all gardening activities, such as tilling, digging, planting, weeding, raking, and mowing.

- Engage in arts and crafts activities, such as building a bird feeder.

- When the weather permits, participate in outdoor exercise, movement, and dance classes.

Auditory-Musical Activities

- When the weather permits, participate in musical activities such as playing instruments, participating in sing-alongs, listening to the radio or audio-cassettes, and joining in outdoor music therapy.

- Participate in a game of musical chairs outside in a courtyard or patio. Practitioners might request that all elder care entertainers incorporate the theme of spring into their musical presentations.

- Watch birds and listen to the sounds of birds.

Interpersonal Activities

- Engage in all group activities, such as gardening and arts and crafts.

- Participate in social interactions, such as creating a group spring collage, caring for a spring garden, or engaging in group discussions and social events.

Intrapersonal Activities

- Engage in spring events and activities that are personally relevant, such as creating a personal book of spring pictures and photographs or planting a garden or window box of flowers.

- Share opinions and memories about the season based on prompts such as "What do you like or what don't you like about spring?"

Naturalistic Activities

- Participate in indoor and outdoor activities that involve caring for plants and animals.

- When weather permits, engage in outdoor activities such as bird-watching, gardening, walking, and sitting.

- Maintain a personal window box of plants.
- Make a bird feeder for outdoor use.

Summer

Usually the summer theme involves sun, outdoors, swimming, lakes, beaches, picnics, boating, Father's Day, the Fourth of July and Labor Day holidays, weddings, and sports such as baseball, golf, and tennis.

Verbal-Linguistic Activities

- Participate in outdoor discussion groups that use summer memories as a focus.
- Engage in group discussion and creative writing activities that use sentence completion formats (e.g., "When I think of summer, I think of . . . " and "In summer I used to . . . ").
- Complete summer-themed crossword puzzles, word finds, and word mazes.
- Create summer memory books using personal photographs from past or current group summer activities.
- Create a summer bulletin board display using summer words (hot, sunny, breezy), photographs, magazine pictures, poems, and creative writings.

Logical-Mathematical Activities

- Create a summer group activity schedule.
- Chart daily summer temperature and weather changes.
- Record and categorize summer events, such as bird watching, maintaining a garden, and attending sports events.
- Organize a picnic basket, an array of Fourth of July decorations, and other summer-related supplies.
- Play games such as puzzles, lotto, and dominoes that involve summer-related themes (plants, flowers, summer sports).

Visual-Spatial Activities

- Create sand art.
- Make baskets out of craft sticks.
- Complete puzzles and coloring books with summer themes (flowers, plants, seashores).

- Create butterfly or flower collages.

- Make flower-chain decorations.

- Create a bulletin board display of summer pictures to prompt recall of summer memories.

- Engage in sponge-art projects with summer themes (summer garden, the sea, boats, a sunny day, a day at the lake, summer showers).

- Sit outdoors and have the person draw what he or she sees. A collection of summer drawings would make a lovely summer-themed bulletin board display.

Tactile-Kinesthetic Activities

- Participate in all outdoor summer sports as well as movement, dance, and social activities (swimming, sponge ball or regular tennis, sponge ball baseball and catch using Velcro mitts, beach volleyball using Velcro paddles and balls, golf, walking, gardening, and lawn care).

- Have individuals with severe Alzheimer's sit outside in a glider or rocking chair to observe others engaged in outdoor activities.

- Participate in summer arts and crafts activities, such as creating sand art, basket weaving, making Fourth of July decorations, finger painting with summer colors, and sculpting clay.

Auditory-Musical Activities

- Watch Fourth of July and Labor Day parades, and listen to songs related to these summer holidays.

- Use summer songfests and karaoke-assisted sing-alongs to encourage individuals to reminisce about summer. Songs such as "Take Me Out to the Ballgame," "In the Good Old Summertime," and "Summertime" should prompt recall. All music and dance activities, such as simple water ballet, should focus on summer themes.

- Listen to audiocassettes or CDs of summer sounds, such as the ocean, rain, and trees blowing in the wind, or of George Winston's musical compositions based on the four seasons of the year.

Interpersonal Activities

- Engage in all theme-related group activities, such as book clubs and group discussions, outdoor sports and gardening activities, summer-oriented arts and crafts, group sing-alongs, picnics, and holiday celebrations.

- Participate in a summer activity planning committee or a group dramatic presentation.

- Take part in a series of theme-related social events, such as "A Summer Fling," a Fourth of July parade, and a group picnic, as well as intergenerational summer activities.

Intrapersonal Activities

- Engage discussions in which the person shares his or her own unique perceptions and memories of summer events. Use "I" in relevant sentence starters and conversation topics (What I like about summer).

- Participate in independent creative writing and crafts projects.

- Take part in an individualized, summer-themed occupational, dance, music, or recreational therapy.

- Create a personalized summer memory book or memory box with personal photographs or items from the past.

- Decorate personal living quarters with relevant summer memorabilia or the person's own crafts.

- If writing skills still exist, write and mail summer postcards to loved ones.

Naturalistic Activities

- Engage in a wide array of nature-related summer activities, such as pet care; butterfly, insect, and stone collecting; gardening; lawn care; bird and animal watching; nature walks; tree pruning; and picking wildflowers.

- Participate in outdoor activities such as swimming, group picnics, sitting, and walking.

- Create and maintain a summer vegetable or flower garden.

- Take part in summer-related arts and crafts and recreational activities that involve plants, animals, insects, and flowers.

- Create a summer weather calendar.

- Collect summer flowers and herbs, dry and press them, and put them in a book.

- Using dried flowers and herbs, make summer potpourri and pressed flower cards, pictures, bookmarks, and placemats.

- Participate in art projects that use birdseeds and sand.

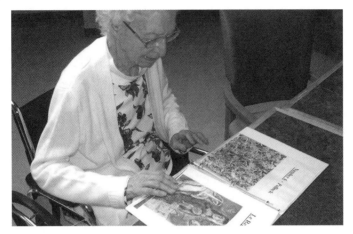

Looking through an interest album of famous painters (intrapersonal/
visual-spatial/verbal-linguistic strengths)

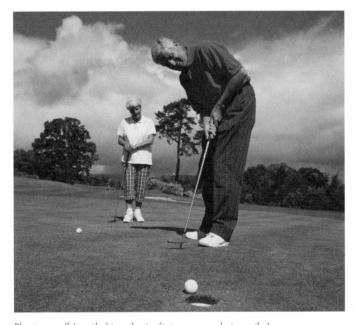

Playing golf (tactile-kinesthetic/interpersonal strengths)

Chapter 4

Modifying Strength-Based Activities to Match the Progression of Dementia

Michelle S. Bourgeois, M.S., Ph.D., CCC-SLP

Individuals with Alzheimer's disease often appear to lose interest in their life-long hobbies as their illness progresses. This may simply be a sign that the complexity of the attempted task is overly challenging, causing stress and frustration, when this same task would have once provided engagement, stimulation, and satisfaction. This chapter provides some specific guidelines and examples of how to analyze the complexity of a task and design activity variations and modifications that will allow a person with Alzheimer's to continue to engage in the task as his or her abilities decline.

The dimensions of a task that can be analyzed and modified to maintain engagement can be categorized as *implicit* and *explicit*. The implicit features of a task require memory processing, including access to long-term, short-term, and procedural memories. Long-term memory of a task is necessary in recognizing that this is a familiar activity. For example, an individual might remember enjoying an activity in his or her youth, or in specific settings, or with certain individuals. Long-term memory is one's personal history of an activity. The accumulation of episodes of engaging in an activity over one's lifetime contributes to skill development and task complexity. A young girl, for example, would have first learned how to thread a needle, then sew a simple stitch, and then hem a simple garment, eventually progressing to complex garments and complex sewing techniques. Throughout her adulthood, her longest history of sewing experience would have been at the most complex level of sewing.

Short-term memory of a task implies, at the time of engagement in the task, the ability to (1) identify the task; (2) recognize what to do at the moment (i.e., know the sequence of rules or steps in the task); (3) know how to keep focused on the task; and (4) understand how others are involved in the task. Because this type of memory (sometimes called *working memory*) is thought to be transient or temporary, and is not stored in long-term memory, it is also thought to be susceptible to interruptions and distractions. For example, when someone engaged in a craft activity hears footsteps, looks up to see a visitor, and is asked what she is doing, she is likely to say she does not know. This is because the new stimuli (i.e., sound of footsteps, sight of visitor, question asked of her) are now being processed in short-term memory and have replaced the memories of the task she was doing.

The procedural memory requirements of a task refer to the actual steps, or process, of doing the task. In considering a lifelong interest, it is to be expected that the task would be well practiced, or overlearned. It would not have to be explained or taught because the person would have done it so frequently that the process is automatic (similar to other overlearned skills, such as eating, walking, and reading). For example, it is common for someone who is handed a memory album to automatically open the book to the first page and continue turning the pages without instruction. Individuals for whom reading is a lifelong experience know instinctively what to do with something that has pages.

Adapting Tasks to Match an Individual's Life Interests with Remaining Competencies

The implicit features of a task are intimately related to its explicit features, or physical characteristics (i.e., size, shape, color, weight, number of parts, and complexity). These explicit dimensions are mediated through the senses (vision, hearing, touch, taste, smell) and can vary systematically. For example, as we age and our vision deteriorates, we use eyeglasses that alter the size and clarity of what we see. As our visual acuity continues to decline, we replace the glasses with progressively stronger lenses. The same can be said for hearing aids. This compensation strategy can be applied to all of the senses and to any characteristic of a task or activity. In the education field, identifying the gradations, or levels or steps, of a task or a stimulus, along a continuum from complex to simple, is called *task analysis*. This process also helps to identify the interrelationships between implicit and explicit features of a task and the ways to modify one feature to compensate for another. The activity examples presented in this chapter are described along a continuum of three levels (from complex to moderate to simple). Level 1 tasks or activities are appropriate for persons with early-stage memory impairment. Level 2 tasks have been modified to reduce complexity for persons with moderate dementia. And level 3 tasks have been simplified to very basic concepts for persons with severe or advanced memory problems.

Consider card playing as an example. Mrs. Smith was an avid bridge player. As a young bride, her husband taught her the game to enjoy at family gatherings. As her skills developed and her confidence grew, she joined a ladies' bridge club, first as a substitute, progressing to regular player, and then serving as captain of her championship duplicate bridge team. She became the preferred instructor of new members, and she read the bridge column in the newspaper religiously. When she retired from the banking industry, she maintained her membership in the club for several years. Over a period of years, she began to miss a meeting once every few months, then once a month, until she had an excuse to miss every occasion. But she spent much of her free time, often hours at a time, playing solitaire. When her family was gathered together, she would occasionally ask to play out a bridge hand. After the bidding had ended, she would be satisfied with one hand and would make an excuse to leave the table. When her grandchildren came to visit, however, she was an enthusiastic player of rummy and Old Maid. Eventually, the cards were put aside. A few years later, Mrs. Smith was rummaging through a drawer and found a deck of cards. She sat down, lovingly fingered the cards, shuffled them a few times, and then dealt them into a pile of reds and a pile of blacks. Later that week, a visiting grandchild shared with her a deck of oversized, large print, number cards. As she inspected each card carefully, she announced its value, "That's a two. That's a six."

Using this example, consider the natural progression of card playing along its dimensions.

Implicit, long-term memory: Mrs. Smith, over the course of her entire life, had developed much skill and experience playing bridge, with her family and her club, informally and in competitions. She could be described as a master, or expert, bridge player and instructor, with significantly more knowledge of the subject (e.g., rules, plays) than most recreational players. Therefore, as she gradually lost cognitive function, she maintained her interest in card playing by simplifying various features. When bridge became too complex a game, she played solitaire (a sequencing task with simple rules). Later she played rummy (a sequencing and matching game) and Old Maid (a matching task). Finally, she separated the cards by color (a discrimination task).

Implicit, short-term memory and procedural memory: When the family played bridge, Mrs. Smith could still play out a hand, though she avoided the more complex bidding process. She was able to remember the mechanics (procedures) of playing out a hand of bridge. She could get enjoyment out of playing rummy and Old Maid with her grandchildren because these games are easier, have simpler rules, and do not take as long to play; distractions have less of an impact when less effort is required to concentrate on a game. Shuffling and dealing cards are overlearned behaviors; Mrs. Smith automatically began shuffling the cards when she felt the weight of them in her hands.

Explicit, sensory-based changes: When shown the large print number cards, Mrs. Smith was able to read the numbers. Changing the print size so she could see the numbers (visual feature) enabled her to read them (an overlearned, procedural memory). No other sensory changes were described in this example.

The examples that follow are only a few of the possible ways to adapt and modify tasks and activities. Each activity contains three levels of complexity for individuals to use as their illness progresses. For individuals living at home, suggestions for participating in social events are included, such as dining in a restaurant, cooking, baking, and attending a barbeque, religious services, and concerts.

Verbal-Linguistic: Scrabble

Level 1

In the game of Scrabble, participants randomly select seven alphabet tiles and attempt to formulate words for the maximum possible points. Words are placed on the game board in a crossword-puzzle format and must intersect with an existing word or words on the board. The game continues until participants' tiles no longer form words to add to the board. The winner is the one who has accumulated the most points. This game requires good vocabulary, spelling, attention, prediction, and working memory skills.

Level 2

To simplify the rules of the game, Scrabble could be played without the game board, eliminating the crossword puzzle aspect of the game. Players can randomly select seven letter tiles and attempt to formulate a word with the letters. Players can take turns placing the word in the middle of the table for all to see; scores can be accumulated by adding the values of each letter tile for each word played. If no word can be formulated, a player can use his or her turn to trade in tiles.

Level 3

Scrabble letter tiles can be used for a word or letter matching game. Word cards can be prepared in advance on topics of interest such as school days (e.g., *pencil, paper, teacher, math, science*), and players uncover tiles from the pile in the middle of the table to match the letters on their card. As a group activity, players can take turns picking a tile and matching it to their card. As a solitary activity, a person can match tiles to letters on the word card until he or she loses interest.

Verbal-Linguistic: Crossword Puzzles

For individuals who enjoyed doing crossword puzzles, this activity can be maintained by selecting puzzles that are fun to do because the person can successfully retrieve the words needed to complete the puzzle. This is done by choosing puzzles that are easier than what the person might have completed before experiencing memory loss; a wide variety of crossword puzzle books are available in bookstores in the adult, preteen, and children's sections. In the later stages of memory loss, computer software programs are available for creating your own crossword puzzles. These programs allow for interest-specific and personalized crossword puzzles to be created that allow the person to practice remembering vocabulary of a favorite hobby or interest, or family members' names. These can be constructed to be at the exact level of complexity or simplicity to be enjoyable for the person.

Logical-Mathematical: Bingo and Lotto Games

Level 1

Bingo is typically played with someone announcing the letter and number combination and players finding the matching number on the card. The first person to cover all numbers on their card along a vertical column, horizontal row, or diagonal is declared the winner. Variations of the game include different patterns of number coverage (e.g., the entire card, the perimeter) and simultaneous playing of multiple cards.

Level 2

Bingo can be modified at the implicit and explicit levels. Cover-the-card bingo reduces the complexity of the rules and the effort required by working memory to remember which variation is being played (horizontal, vertical, diagonal, etc.). Displaying the letter and number combinations on a large board or on bingo cards can reduce the impact of short-term memory loss; having to remember what someone says is more difficult than having information in a visual format that can be monitored repeatedly until the matching task is complete.

Level 3

Bingo can be further simplified by increasing the diversity of the items to be matched. Because there is redundancy in number tasks, regular bingo requires good attention and discrimination skills for success. For example, determining "34" from "43" can be a difficult discrimination. Lotto games that have a similar structure to bingo (i.e., a card with rows and columns of items), but include interesting picture stimuli, can maintain a person's engagement in game playing at a simpler level of complexity. Lotto games can be designed to overcome sensory deficits. For example, an 8-by-8-inch lotto card can be divided into an 8-by-8 array of 64 squares, or a 4-by-4 array of 16 squares, or a 2-by-2 array of 4 squares, thereby increasing the visual size of the pictured item and decreasing the complexity of the game. The topic of the lotto game can be anything of interest to the participants (e.g., clothing, foods, animals, musical instruments, golf equipment, famous paintings).

Visual-Spatial and Tactile-Kinesthetic: In the Kitchen

Level 1

For the housewife and mother who has spent a lifetime preparing meals for her family, memory problems can create many frustrating and embarrassing situations. Some early signs of memory loss are forgetting specific ingredients in a familiar recipe and creating something that does not taste or look quite right. Loss of interest in cooking and baking can signal underlying insecurities about memory problems. Memory aids in the form of written recipes, weekly menu planning, and shopping lists are important tools to use in ways that do not accentuate the memory problem, and instead support the creation of delicious meals. Family members can approach this task by emphasizing the person's cooking skills and the need for these skills to be transferred to future generations. For example, solicit the individual's assistance in documenting favorite family recipes. Make a "Family Favorites" cookbook, with step-by-step instructions and detailed lists of ingredients. The person will likely be very proud to give the family cookbook as a gift to his or her grandchildren.

Provide a weekly menu template and find a time to discuss and plan together a healthy menu of breakfast, lunch, and dinner foods; this can be particularly enjoyable for the person if the discussion allows for reminiscing about specific funny or memorable times related to food preparation. "Remember when you were going to teach me how to make bread and we forgot to add the yeast, so we spent hours and hours watching the dough just sit there?" Once the weekly menu is planned, the next step is to create the shopping list for needed items. Start with making a list of items needed for each day's menu, then checking the refrigerator and pantry for the items, crossing off the list the ones that are present and circling the items needed to purchase. Keep the list in a visible location in the kitchen until it is time to go shopping.

Level 2

As memory problems increase, a gradual change in routine can ease the transition from the person being solely responsible for the cooking and meal preparation to being involved in the process. Family members can plan to assume responsibility for the cooking and shopping, while requesting advice from the person about how to do these tasks. Meal planning, shopping, and cooking together allow the person to feel as though he or she is still performing these tasks, while the family member ensures that the tasks are executed correctly and safely. If a "Family Favorites" cookbook has been compiled, selecting and following the recipes while cooking will ensure a successful result. Family recipes usually create enough food for a family of four or more; if the person is single or living with a spouse, the leftovers can be packaged for future meals. It is important to label each container with the contents and the date of preparation. Incorporating children into meal preparation activities is another way to convey the importance of the knowledge and skills the person has to share with future generations. The person can be encouraged to show a child how to knead bread dough or how to clean and prepare a chicken for roasting.

Level 3

When an individual can no longer prepare food independently, family members can ensure that this important lifetime role is maintained and celebrated by creating opportunities for the person to assist with meal preparation and cooking or baking but no longer be responsible for the preparatory steps. Asking the person to stir the cookie batter, knead the bread dough, or slice the mushrooms keeps him or her engaged in the tasks and feeling productive. Asking the person to help with washing or drying the dishes, or setting the table, or judging if the chicken is browned enough maintains her identity as the expert in matters related to the roles of mother and homemaker. When these tasks become too challenging, simply sitting in the kitchen, smelling the cooking odors, or handling the vegetables stimulates memories that are meaningful and satisfying.

Tactile-Kinesthetic: Golf

Level 1

Golf can continue to be a satisfying physical activity once competitive tournament play is no longer feasible. The following modifications often occur naturally: playing a shorter game (9 holes instead of 18), using a golf cart between fairways, and noting each individual's score for each hole after completing each hole or keeping no score at all, and allowing players to choose the course of play.

Level 2

Golf can be minimized to either putting or driving by playing golf on the putting green or the driving range. This eliminates the layer of complexity that the rules of the game impose and serves to focus attention on one skill at a time. Putting and driving can also be limited in duration to conserve energy and reduce fatigue. Indoor putting games that have automatic ball return can also be an enjoyable alternative.

Level 3

A variety of games with golf themes can be developed to engage the individual, including golf bingo using a game board with golf terms in categories (e.g., clubs, golf bag, cart, score card, flag). Individuals can also play golf lotto using a game board that includes pictures of golf items. Sorting golf tees by size and color and sorting the golf balls by color or brand might also prove enjoyable.

Auditory-Musical: Classical Music ▬▬▬▬▬

Level 1

Classical musicians, those individuals who were proficient in playing a musical instrument at some point in years past, should maintain this overlearned behavior for many years. These individuals typically can be easily coaxed to perform familiar songs from memory, without the need to read the music. They often enjoy reading and playing simpler versions of familiar music from children's music books. Typically these books have fewer but larger notes per page.

Individuals who once enjoyed professional concerts may find it overly challenging to keep their attention focused on a lengthy piece of music and may fall asleep or become restless. Community or school recitals can often be an enjoyable, and shorter, alternative. Some musical genres, like musicals and musical theatre, are well suited to people with memory challenges; the quick pace of the action, musical selections, and change in actors and scenes can keep the person engaged in the production. Reviewing the written program before the start of the show can help to remind the person of the story and names of characters. Similarly, rereading the list of songs in the first act, and the ones to come in the second act, can stimulate conversation about the show.

Level 2

Classical music lovers may have a wealth of untapped musical knowledge that can be used to design engaging activities that go beyond listening to familiar

music. These individuals might enjoy reading about music. Articles about famous musicians, different instruments, and other musical topics can be used
for individual pleasure or group discussions. Magazines for children, such as
Clavier's Piano Explorer, are ideal sources of elementary-level materials that include activities such as word searches.

Individuals with auditory-musical intelligence might also enjoy music games. Commercially available children's games on music topics can
be appropriate as designed, or adapted as necessary. There are music trivia
games, instrument–sound matching games, and composer–genre games. For
example, one instrument game includes a game board and individual instrument cards to arrange in a typical orchestra configuration. These same instrument
cards can be sorted by categories (e.g., woodwinds, strings, brass). Activity personnel can create trivia questions about a show or concert that was attended by
a group of residents; the program from the show or concert is a good source of
pictures and information for the trivia game.

Level 3

Music games and activities can be adapted further to maintain interest and
engagement. Musical bingo and lotto games can be constructed for a variety
of musical topics. Bingo cards can be constructed with categories such as com-
posers, instruments, song titles, and music notation written along the top row
of the bingo card. Examples of each category are written in the appropriate
down column. Pictures of instruments, equipment, musical notes, and com-
posers can be used for lotto cards.

Simple instruments to play, such as harmonicas, triangles, and tambou-
rines, can be the focus of a group play-along activity. Other instruments might
be more appropriate for touching and reminiscing activities (e.g., violin, banjo,
trumpet, and accordion). In addition, song identification games, in which song
clips are listened to, then the title is chosen from a list of potential titles (or
artists, or albums), are very popular group activities. Individuals might also
enjoy small musical instrument puzzles of 6 to 24 pieces.

Interpersonal and Verbal-Linguistic: Group Discussion and Book Clubs

Level 1

The success of a discussion group or a book club is often related to the level
of interest the participants have in the topic, the richness of their own experiences with the topic, and the skills of the facilitator to ensure all participants
have opportunities to share their thoughts. Interviewing the participants and
their family members and reviewing their life story should provide a wealth of

information from which to select engaging topics, including preferred types of reading materials (e.g., fiction, nonfiction, autobiography, best sellers). Topics common to most group participants usually lead to more interaction and discussion. The use of objects, reading materials, and pictures as topic prompts can help to maintain focus on the featured topic. Discussion groups that follow a structured format (e.g., participants read a high-interest, large-print reading selection and then answer question prompts to identify the main topic, characters, action, timeline, and subplots) are often maintained over longer periods of time because of the predictability, familiarity, and comfort level the structure provides.

Level 2

At this level, more explicit prompts may be required to maintain attention to a topic of conversation and to elicit personal long-term memories. Written prompts in the form of topic headings, category headings, and questions reduce the short-term memory effort required to keep the topic in mind while trying to remember something related and personal to share. Chalkboards or erasable-marker boards are useful for visual aids. Writing in large print and using colored markers can also provide extra visual cues. Reading materials in large-print format are available for many genres of reading materials. The Internet is a good source for book club discussion guides and suggested questions and topics for specific books.

Level 3

When interpersonal interaction is a person's strength, simply sitting next to other people or being in the same room with others is an expression of this personal trait. Conversation at this level can be maintained using appropriate prompts for personal information, such as personalized cue cards, memory book pages, labeled photographs, and special objects or collections of items. The contents of a woman's purse can elicit much discussion and facilitate retrieval of long-term memories. For example, a mirrored compact might lead to a discussion of powdering one's nose or other favorite cosmetics. A gentleman's cigar box might contain a variety of items that spark memories of a prior military career (e.g., combat medals, expired military identification card, dog tags). One person's treasures can promote discussion of others' favorite things. Sharing pictures of grandchildren is a popular conversation starter. Make sure the pictures have the child's name in large print for everyone to read.

Book clubs can continue successfully at this stage when the reading materials are large print and simplified text presented in short paragraphs that group participants can take turns reading aloud. Written questions that refer directly to the text allow participants to successfully find the answers to the questions in the paragraph, and open-ended questions can be used to elicit personal memories related to the story. Several series of dementia-specific reading materials are available for purchase (e.g., Hearthstone Readers); activity personnel, however, can prepare materials specific to the interests of their clients and duplicate copies for each participant.

Interpersonal: Social Events ▨

Level 1

Social events in public places present challenges for a person with memory loss. It is expected that he or she will be able to participate in conversations, display socially appropriate behaviors, and inhibit socially inappropriate behavior when going out to eat at a restaurant or a friend's backyard barbecue, shopping, or participating in a religious service. Often, however, a person with Alzheimer's may need memory supports to put to use these lifelong interpersonal skills. Planning for these events before they happen can prevent unexpected confusion, embarrassing memory lapses, and undesired behaviors. Some ideas for planning include reviewing a calendar and other important details about an upcoming event or outing, such as the names of people who will likely be in attendance or the possible menu selections. A calendar in a variety of formats is an important memory support. A large format, dry-erase board that displays each day of the month is useful for writing down all appointments, social events, and outings. This board should be hung in a prominent location in the home where the person is likely to walk past it many times during the day. Review the calendar together at routine times of the day, such as before or after meals. It is important to discuss the events that are planned and ones that have occurred to help keep information about those events activated in memory and more likely to be remembered. Pocket calendars or planners are also recommended so that they can be checked wherever and whenever the person needs to remember a daily plan.

Word-finding problems that are increasingly common with advancing age can be particularly embarrassing and can cause a person to become fearful of social situations. Planning for social situations can help to address this challenge, including reviewing the names of people who likely will be in attendance, thinking of things to talk about and questions to ask other people, and anticipating what food items will be on the menu. A simple notebook is a useful memory tool in keeping lists of names of people in various social groups (e.g., "People from church," "Former work colleagues," "My doctor's office"). Before a specific event, the list of names can be read, activating them in the person's working memory and increasing the likelihood that they will be remembered at the time of a social interaction with the individuals who are listed. The notebook can have other lists or categories of words or topics of conversation that can be reviewed prior to an event to reduce anxiety about potential memory lapses.

Level 2

Memory aids that provide access to information that is typically difficult to retrieve in the moment need to be with the person when he or she is in social situations. If a calendar, or planner, has been incorporated into the daily routine, then a pocket-sized version needs to be carried by the person when he or she is away from home. Some planners include Notes sections where lists of names, conversation topics, or other words can be written. If the person seems reluctant or embarrassed to refer to the planner during social situations, spend 5 minutes in the car reviewing the information with him or her before an event. This can increase the person's confidence in his or her social skills. The person can also take comfort in knowing that the words or names he or she might need are close at hand, in his or her pocket or purse.

Level 3

As problems with memory increase, memory aids may need some simple modifications to remain useful in social situations. To enhance conversations with others, a small notebook with pictures and short sentences or phrases can allow the person to be able to talk about important topics with others. Encourage family members and friends to ask the person to show them the notebook and use it to talk to the person about the information it contains. Prepare a list of recent events for the person to talk about with others; another list could have suggested questions for the person to ask.

In some restaurants, picture menus are available to facilitate food selections. Discussing in advance what to expect in terms of food selections, circumstances of the event (outdoor barbecue or formal wedding reception), and people in attendance will lessen potential confusion and anxiety about the situation. Write short scripts for common conversational interactions and practice them in advance of the event. For example, at an event where the person will be meeting unfamiliar people, an acceptable script would be: "It's nice to meet you." "My name is (name). Where are you from?" Anticipate usual questions that would be asked in these situations and practice responding ("What kind of dressing would you like on your salad?" "I'd like blue cheese, thank you.").

In social situations that require silence, such as church services or weddings, it is helpful to have something for the person to read or look at if his or her attention wanders and he or she forgets to remain quiet. An interest album or a small memory book (as described above) can help to keep the person engaged in looking at something interesting during the event. An index card with a simple message ("Shhh . . . no talking now" or "We'll be leaving in 5 minutes") can be shown to a person who looks as though he or she might be about to talk aloud. For lengthy events it may be preferable to have someone sit with the person in another room where he or she can talk and do activities.

Large family gatherings, holiday parties, or other social events with many people can often be overwhelming, noisy, and overstimulating. It is wise to plan for quiet interludes for the person to interact one-on-one with a favorite grandchild or niece in another room or away from the larger group. Have the person's memory book or interest albums available for sharing during these special times.

Intrapersonal: Memory Books

Level 1

Having an illustrated biography of one's life can be most comforting, especially when awareness of memory lapses is acute. Commercially available grandmother's and grandfather's books can help an individual to organize and document on paper the many memories he or she would want family members to hand down through the generations. Each page prompts the person to write about a specific time in his or her life or a particularly important event, or to provide some words of wisdom about a topic. There is usually blank space for photos or drawings, should the person want to complement the text. Some people are overwhelmed by the task of completing a book such as this, in which case family members can use the book as a guide for questions and topics, tape-record themselves interviewing the person, and later transcribe the conversation onto the relevant pages. The individual appreciates this gift. When blank pages remain in the book, the person can add his or her thoughts during quiet moments of reflection.

Scrapbooking is a popular pastime that incorporates many of the ideas of documenting important events in a person's life. Memory books can be made in the form of scrapbooks, using a variety of artifacts, including photographs and memorabilia from special events. Family members can assist with purchasing supplies, guiding the layout and selection of photographs, mementos, and decorative borders and suggesting captions to capture the essential details of the event for later review. It is important to include written captions in the scrapbook so that it can be a used as a memory book in the later stages when the person will have increasing difficulty retrieving words. When the captions are written in the person's own handwriting, they are more likely to accept what is written as truthful and accurate. This can be especially useful in the later stages when memory problems intensify and the person can be suspicious of what others tell him or her. Having important facts about an individual's life written in his or her own handwriting can be a great comfort to the person and an important tool for family and caregivers to use in helping to relieve the person's anxieties and fears that occur with memory loss.

Level 2

Family members and friends should take the initiative to make a memory book, or a memory scrapbook, for the individual. It is important, however, to involve the person in making the memory book. Be sure to ask him or her to help select the pictures, as those will likely elicit the most conversation. When making the book, start off with biographical information about the person (e.g., his or her name, date and location of birth, names of parents, siblings, and spouse), written in large print letters and with one simple statement per page. Some books have entire sections about the person's current living situation and activities of daily living (e.g., "I live at Quiet Oaks Senior Apartments," "I wake up at 8:00 in the morning," "I spend time with my friends, Mabel and Helen."). Most books have some pages that show the person's interests and hobbies. It can also be very reassuring to have information in the book that is of a sensitive nature (e.g., "My husband died of cancer in 1989 and is buried in Woodlawn Cemetery"), as well as information that is difficult to remember (e.g., "My pension check is automatically deposited in the bank every month").

Level 3

Memory books can be modified to maintain a person's effectiveness in spite of his or her declining abilities. For an individual whose illness necessitates institutional care, a memory book needs to be lightweight, portable, and conducive to frequent use. This can be done by writing the most important information on index cards and attaching them to the person's wheelchair or his or her clothing via a belt, necklace, or pocket. Before moving to institutional care, it is advisable to add pages to an existing memory book or make a separate book about the person's home. Pictures of the outside and inside of the home, the different rooms, and the person's favorite belongings can help him or her to remember home. The final pages should explain and illustrate the new living arrangement in positive terms (e.g., "I now live at Quiet Oaks Senior Apartments," "I feel safe here," "The friendly staff takes care of my laundry and housework").

Interest albums are memory books, or scrapbooks, about specific hobbies and interests that can also be particularly engaging and comforting. A gardener might enjoy an album about flower gardens that displays large, colorful pictures of the different types of flowers he or she grew. Typed, large-print labels for each flower will help the person to remember the names of the flowers. A sports lover might enjoy an entire album about football. Magazines are good sources of action shots of football players from various teams. The captions in this sort of album might include "The Washington Redskins," "The Pittsburgh Steelers," and "A great catch!" Activity directors can engage residents in making scrapbook pages about specific events, holidays, or other themes to add to a memory book or scrapbook, using magazine pictures, arts and crafts supplies, recycled greeting cards, scraps of gift wrapping paper and ribbon, pieces of fabric, or other tangibles. Captions describing the event (e.g., "Our Valentine's Day Party," or "Our Trip to the Art Museum") can be typed on a computer and printed in multiples, one for each member of the group to paste onto a page in his or her book.

Naturalistic: Fishing ▨

Level 1

Fishing may be one of the more solitary activities people enjoy as a hobby. Yet some avid fishermen enjoy sharing the joys of this quiet sport with a friend or family member, especially a grandchild. Keep in mind how the individual enjoyed this hobby throughout his or her life when designing activity modifications. When personal safety during solitary fishing becomes a concern, a family member or friend should offer to take the person fishing at a familiar location. Ample time should be devoted to reviewing and selecting the necessary equipment and supplies, preparing the tackle box, discussing and getting the bait, and loading it into the car. Expect that the fishing excursion will be of shorter duration than in the past because of short-term memory and attention constraints. The individual may not appear as patient with the lack of fishing success as in the past. If the fish are not biting, the individual might want to move along to the next favorite spot. The mechanics of fishing (e.g., baiting the hook, casting, and reeling) should be no problem because they are overlearned skills.

Level 2

Once the lack of attention and patience begins to interfere with fishing enjoyment, use the following modifications to maintain the individual's engagement in the activity.

- Fishing in a stocked pond ensures rapid success in obtaining a fish and ensures satisfaction and pride. Once a fish has been caught, the cleaning tasks can make for a complete outing. Conversation during the cleaning can focus on the size, feel, and parts of the fish (vocabulary stimulation), and then lead to cooking the fish at home. This variation of the typical fishing outing is shorter and more focused on accomplishing the entire range of related activities.

- Games that accentuate the solitary nature of fishing are often engaging for the fisherman. Fishing magazines are good sources of pictures and ideas for simple bingo, lotto, and sorting and matching games that can be completed individually. Categories such as types of fish (bass, trout, salmon, cod, catfish); locations (lake, stream, ocean, freshwater, saltwater); size (tiny, small, medium, large); fish parts (head, tail, body, eye, mouth, fins, gills, scales); equipment (pole, line, hook, bait, bucket); and lures (dry flies, poppers, spinners, plastic plugs) can provide many words and pictures for cards.

- A simple magnet fishing game can be made with a bucket, a dowel with string and magnet on the end, and fish pictures, each with a paper clip or magnetic strip attached. Once caught, the fish can be sorted by different categories (size, type, location).

Level 3

Outdoor fishing activities can be modified to be spectator sports at this level. When a friend invites the individual to go fishing, the preparations can be abbreviated; a fishing hat, tackle box, and pole may be sufficient equipment to load into the vehicle. Select a fishing location guaranteed to attract other fishermen so that the individual can watch others fishing. Fishing from a dock may be the ideal location for walking back and forth and seeing the fish others have caught.

To maintain an interest in fishing when confined to the indoors, engage the individual in touching and feeling activities. A tackle box with a variety of safe fishing gear, such as lures, a roll of fishing line, bobbers, spinners, rubber worms, or a fishing hat with lures attached, and an expired fishing license can keep someone engaged for a long time.

Naturalistic: Gardening ▰▰▰▰▰▰▰▰▰▰▰▰▰▰

Level 1

Gardening (vegetable or flower gardening or yard maintenance) may have been a solitary activity that an individual enjoyed throughout much of his or her lifetime. At this level, it is important to support the individual's continued independence in doing these activities by using visual cues to remind the person to do specific activities. For example, there can be an entry on a calendar that says "Rake the back yard" or "Trim the rose bush by the garage." A "honey-do" list on the refrigerator that lists multiple yard tasks can be checked off as each task is completed. Placing relevant items for completing gardening tasks in plain view can gently remind the person to do the task, such as a rake and an empty leaf bag near the back door or a basket and clippers on the kitchen table for harvesting beans or tomatoes.

Level 2

At this stage, there may be an increased need for supervision of gardening and lawn maintenance tasks in order for the person to maintain sufficient attention to accomplish the tasks, and sometimes there are safety concerns. It is always desirable to find ways to maintain a person's dignity and expertise for a task by asking if he or she would show you, or a grandchild, how to do the task. Putting yourself, or the grandchild, in the role of helper and/or learner allows the person to remain in charge of the activity, while you are monitoring his or her safety and the execution of the task. Planning activities, such as designing the planting of a garden, choosing which vegetables or shrubs to purchase and when to plant them, are other potentially enjoyable ways to maintain engagement in a lifelong outdoor interest. Gardening magazines and catalogs are useful visual cues for helping the person to make choices for future garden or yard projects.

Level 3

Taking a walk through a yard or garden is an important way to access vocabulary and important memories, especially if you describe for the person what you see along the way ("There's the forever rose bush; looks like it needs to be pruned; the roses were such a vivid red this year"). Raised flower beds provide opportunities to use a trowel to dig holes for transplanting flowers, planting seeds, or patting down the dirt around a plant. Other enjoyable activities outdoors include picking flowers in the summer or gathering a bouquet of colorful fall leaves. When the weather gets cooler, indoor gardening activities can include transplanting houseplants from small to larger containers, arranging artificial flowers in vases, looking at gardening magazines, catalogs, or a personalized interest album about the person's own garden or favorite flowers. Craft activities that involve coloring, cutting/pasting/assembling flower or vegetable themed pictures, greeting cards, placemats, or table settings might also be enjoyable.

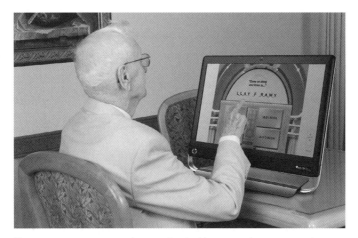

Playing a computer word game (verbal-linguistic/intrapersonal strengths).

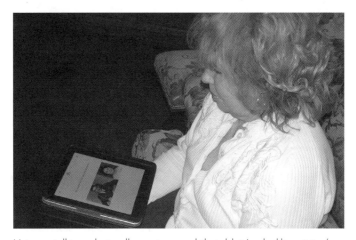

Using a talking photo album via a mobile tablet (verbal-linguistic/intrapersonal strengths).

Chapter 5

New Roles for Technology in Strength-Based Interventions

◼︎

Joan L. Green, M.A., CCC-SLP

Technology's potential to have a positive impact on the lives of individuals with Alzheimer's disease and other forms of dementia has grown exponentially in recent years. Everyone deserves to be exposed to the many benefits technology has to offer—even those with dementia. As baby boomers age and younger generations are more tech savvy, technology is no longer perceived as a luxury, but more as an expectation. The use of tablets and smartphones as well as other cutting-edge devices is in its infancy among the older adult population. There are, however, many affordable technologies that can greatly enhance the overall quality of life for individuals with mild to significant cognitive deficits. Some technologies are more appropriate in the mild stage of Alzheimer's while others are more suitable in the moderate and severe stages. The majority of the products mentioned in this chapter can typically be used with individuals at various stages of cognitive impairment; the task and expectations need to change depending on the goal of the activity.

Persons with dementia, as well as their caregivers, friends, and family, can benefit from technology-based activities that are adapted to their unique abilities and interests and in which the focus of the activity is enjoyment through engagement. Previous experience with items such as a computer, tablet (iPad, Kindle, Galaxy), or other technologies is not necessary in order for the person to benefit from strength-based interventions coupled with technology.

This chapter is not meant to be an exhaustive review of all the technology tools available, but rather a sampling of the many types of technologies available to facilitate activities. An emphasis is placed on empowering the reader to be creative in selecting tech-based activities and using them in a way to promote success and happiness for a person with dementia. Many resources are provided so that readers can continue to learn about cutting-edge technologies as they become available. The applications, or apps, listed in this chapter generally refer to iOS apps, which work on Apple products such as an iPad. Many of the apps, however, are also available for use on devices that use the Android operating system. Product features, pricing, and platforms—especially in the technology world—are ever evolving and, therefore, Web sites are provided for reference. Many developers who produced products described in this chapter have plans to further develop their products to increase their compatability with a wider variety of devices so that more people are able to benefit from them.

Benefits of Technology

Technology can greatly enrich the lives of individuals who use it. When implemented effectively, the benefits of incorporating technology into strength-based programming to help people with dementia include the following:

- Distract from anxiety or pain.

- Lessen depression or apathy.

- Reduce or eliminate fears (e.g., practicing steps in a task or viewing a video to prepare for a future event).

- Increase engagement with others.

- Enhance recall.

- Improve enjoyment of "the here and now."

- Provide an outlet for creativity.

- "Visit" places that may be out of reach or inaccessible (e.g., a museum or distant location).

- "Participate" in sports that may be physically challenging (e.g., tennis or bowling).

- Read text that may be difficult to see due to poor vision.

- Communicate better when unable to recall words or speak clearly.

- Stimulate interaction with family and friends.

- Minimize feelings of isolation when seeing and communicating with people from a distance.

- Engage with younger people in tech-based intergenerational activities.

- Use visual supports for learning new skills to maximize independence (e.g., walking, eating, and taking medicine).

Getting Started

The following are important guidelines to keep in mind as you begin to use technology during activities with people who have dementia:

- A touch screen with direct selection is typically the easiest and most intuitive form of technology to use. Many seniors, especially those with cognitive challenges, have a difficult time using a selecting device such as a mouse or trackball. A tablet with a touch screen is a great way to start. Some individuals may find a stylus is easier to use than a finger.

- Activities should be enjoyable and engaging.

- It is often very challenging for the person with dementia to learn new games, so familiar ones with a limited number of rules or steps are usually the most successful.

- A simple interface is best. It is good to start with large pictures and text as well as a format that is visually appealing.

- Content should be senior friendly. This can be challenging because many products that are cognitively simplistic are produced for children. It is critical that the material not be too juvenile for or insulting to the person. There are times, however, when seniors are amused by the more juvenile content and enjoy using materials created for younger children.

- As discussed throughout this book, an activity selected for intervention should be based on the individual's current strengths and abilities and be tailored to meet the person's needs and interests.

- Create a positive interaction with the product using visually based supportive teaching methods to facilitate success.

- When working with individuals who have severe cognitive impairments, it is helpful to initially have the person watch a practitioner or family member independently use the device app or feature and then slowly start to help the person move his or her hand to touch the screen and cause something to happen. An example of technologies that are appropriate for individuals who have severely impaired cognition that are listed later in this chapter include

    - ❖ soothing music (listed in the music intelligence section),

    - ❖ family pictures with voice output (listed in the visual intelligence section),

    - ❖ visual cause-and-effect products (listed in the kinesthetic intelligence section).

Types of Technologies to Consider

There are many types of technology that when matched appropriately to the needs of the individual can be very helpful. Some of the products are produced specifically to help people with disabilities, while others can help people with dementia overcome barriers to performing everyday tasks. Individuals can use special software, such as watching video demonstrations on a tablet, to practice specific skills. Other technologies, such as the Livescribe Pen (which records audio as a person writes with a special pen on special paper) and text to speech (which reads text aloud), both described later in this chapter, can help the user compensate for areas of weakness. There are technologies that when properly configured can be used independently by the individual, while other products require interaction with a caregiver to facilitate targeted behaviors. Some technologies need customization to be appropriate, while others cannot be customized but can be used in different ways with different people to create a great activity. The type of technology that is used needs to be re-evaluated as a person's cognitive abilities change. It is for this reason that the Informal Geriatric Strength-Based Inventory, described earlier in Chapter 2, should be used throughout the disease progression to assess an individual's current competencies.

Accessibility

Many accessibility options are available for Web browsers, desktop and laptop computers, tablets, and software that will enlarge text, make a keyboard easier to use (e.g., if an individual has a tremor), allow sequential rather than simultaneous keystrokes (e.g., control/alt/delete), and offer text to speech or speech to text, and so forth. Video tutorials to assist a caregiver or clinician in setting up these options for an individual with dementia are available on the following Web sites:

- Microsoft (http://www.microsoft.com/enable)

- Apple (http://www.apple.com/accessibility)

- Google (http://www.google.com/accessibility)

- Firefox (http://www.accessfirefox.org)

Mobile Touchscreen Devices

Mobile touchscreen devices, such as tablets and smartphones that have become increasingly available and affordable, are the best types of technology to use with individuals who have dementia. Many play music and movies with high-quality sound and offer high-resolution touchscreens that are increasingly intuitive and that show clear, vibrant images. They are also very light and portable yet large enough for individuals with impaired vision or limited dexterity to use. Tablets and smartphones offer accessible features and many helpful built-in options, and an ever-growing number of apps are available to run on either type of device. Tablets and smartphones run different operating systems than desktop and laptop computers. A few of the best options for tablets are as follows:

- iPad by Apple (http://www.store.apple.com/us/browse/home/shop_ipad)

- Nexus 7 by Google (https://play.google.com)

- Surface by Microsoft (http://www.microsoft.com/surface)

- Samsung Galaxy by Samsung (http://www.samsung.com/galaxy)

Tablets and Smartphones generally have touch technology. Users can use a finger or stylus pen to select items. Most offer functionality that can help to engage individuals with dementia in activities. The use of visual supports is critical to the successful implementation of activities, whether as part of programming or daily life. It is difficult for individuals with cognitive impairments to focus and understand fleeting auditory inputs, such as spoken instructions.

In my work as a clinician, I primarily use an iPad and Apple apps found via iTunes (http://www.itunes.com) with most individuals who have dementia. All of the apps listed in this chapter can be used with iPads, and some, but not all, are also available for devices with other operating systems, such as Android or Microsoft. If you have a device that runs another operating system (such as a Kindle, Galaxy, or Surface), you will need to explore further to determine exactly which apps are compatible with your device. Not all Android devices are compatible with all Android apps, because the operating system is an "open source" and is available to the public at large and not regulated in the way that Apple products are. For more information about Android apps, visit the Google Play Store at https://play.google.com/store. The following is a sampling of the types of functionality that can be used with an iPad and other tablets to engage people with dementia:

- **Calendar:** Use calendars to help individuals

    ❖ stay organized and remember past events as well as plan upcoming events;

    ❖ prompt conversations, assist with recall of information, and practice language skills;

    ❖ have access to calendar information at all times by syncing the information on multiple devices;

    ❖ coordinate schedules with family members and caregivers.

In the mild stages of dementia it may be an appropriate activity to help the individual enter items into a calendar by speaking or typing. In more severe stages, someone else can enter the information. Basic visually appealing calendars with pictures and voice output can be used to assist the individual with memory, orientation, and communication.

- **Calendar.google.com:** This online calendar is very helpful and can be shared by family members and caregivers who can enter information online and sync it with a tablet and smartphone. It is currently the easist and most reliable intermediary to sync calendars on different operating systems and devices.

- **Visual Schedule Planner:** An app offered by Good Karma Applications, this visually appealing calendar for the iPad integrates pictures, video, and voice output and is customizable. Events that require more support can be linked to an "activity schedule" or "video clip" to help model the task for the individual. Timers, checklists, reminders, and notes also can be added.

- **Cozi Family Organizer:** An app offered by Cozi Group, Inc. (http://www.cozi.com), this calendar is compatible with most computers, tablets, and phones and can be used to coordinate many members of a family who share information. It offers many helpful features, such as a place for journal entries and shopping lists. It can be accessed from any online computer, tablet, or smartphone.

- **Contact Tools:** Just about all tablets and smartphones come preloaded with tools to help organize a person's contact information for family, friends, and other acquaintances. Information can be entered in a way to facilitate recall of information as needed. For instance, the names of a friend's children can be entered for future reference. Also, multiple tags or searchable terms can be used, such as "doctor." If the individual cannot remember a doctor's name, he or she can search for "doctor" and all of the contacts that have that word in their entry will be shown. The following apps take contact tools a step further:

  - ❖ **Bump:** Share contact information, photos, videos, and files by bumping two smartphones together. (Bump Technologies, Inc., http://www.bu.mp)

  - ❖ **CardMunch:** Converts information from a business card into a contact for a smartphone or tablet by taking a picture of the card. (LinkedIn Corporation, http://www.cardmunch.com)

  - ❖ **Unus Tactus:** Turns a cell phone into a one-touch photo dialer. There is a large red "help" button that can be programmed as an alert as needed when an individual leaves a designated geographic radius. It can be customized to send alert emails to specified people and include a map of where the phone is located. (Ashley Alliano, http://www.unustactus.com)

- **Games:** An individual can enjoy playing alone or with others to stimulate cognition. Many gaming apps are listed in the verbal-linguistic and logical-mathematical sections of this chapter.

- **Still and video cameras:** View people as you speak to them from a distance with an app such as Skype or FaceTime, or take still pictures to help with communication and memory. Actions can be videotaped to assist with memory of events and to help learn new skills.

- **Photos and customizable talking books:** View pictures of family and friends as part of a reminiscence program and to help with speaking and understanding. Just about all computers as well as mobile tablets can be used to look at pictures. Customized talking photo albums can be a great resource for activities. Activities can focus on creating the stories or talking pictures or they can be used to help the individual interact with others and learn new skills with step-by-step visual and auditory instructions, choice making, and personal information. Many ways that photos can be used to help a wide variety of individuals are presented near the end of the this chapter. There are many special apps as well as devices to add text, categorize information, and add sound or special effects, including the following:

  ❖ Pictello, by AssistiveWare (http://www.assistiveware.com/product/pictello)

  ❖ Tapikeo, by by Jean-Eudes Lepelletier (http://www.tapikeo.com)

  ❖ Talking Photo Album, by EnableMart (http://www.enablemart.com/Catalog/Basic-Communicators/Talking-Photo-Album)

- **Keyboards:** Most people find larger keyboards easier to use when typing information to help with memory or when sending an email to a friend. Bluetooth keyboards can be used with iPads, and larger keyboards can connect via a USB (universal drive adapter) to other tablets, a laptop, or desktop computer.

- **Microphones:** Dictate notes as well as record what others say to help recall information, such as a doctor's recommendations at a medical appointment. Newer tablets and smartphones offer voice dictation for any app that uses a keyboard. When a microphone appears in the keyboard on the screen, users can speak into the tablet or phone instead of typing via a keyboard and their words will be entered as text and can be seen on the device screen. There are also apps and devices as well as built-in accessibility software features that will record audio as notes are written. Examples of these all-in-one notepad and voice recorders, include

- ❖ AudioNote app, by Luminant Software, Inc.

- ❖ Notability app, by Ginger Labs

- ❖ Livescribe Smartpen, by Livescribe.com. This is a pen with a built-in optical scanner that is used with special paper to sync notes with audio.

- ❖ Microsoft Word for Mac, by Microsoft. The ability to record audio as notes are typed is an included feature of the software.

- **Maps:** Find locations to assist with communication or to obtain help with navigation. Locate where people are from or want to go and practice giving verbal directions or talking about past trips.

  - ❖ Google Maps app or Maps.google.com, by Google. Can be used online or as an app.

  - ❖ Waze app, by Waze Inc. Can be used on a tablet or smartphone.

  - ❖ Mapquest.com or MapQuest app, by AOL. Can be used online or as an app.

- **Movies and TV shows:** View favorite TV shows and movies on a computer, tablet, or smartphone. Content can be streamed online from sites or downloaded onto a device. Old movies and TV shows are readily available. Musicals, nature documentaries, and sitcoms provide a great source of entertainment without the need to process a complicated plot.

  - ❖ http://www.hulu.com

  - ❖ http://www.netflix.com

  - ❖ http://www.play.google.com

  - ❖ http://www.itunes.com

  - ❖ http://www.youtube.com

- **Virtual field trips:** Individuals who have difficulty traveling often enjoy feeling as if they were in a different place by viewing a virtual tour.

  - ❖ http://www.virtualfreesites.com/museums.museums.html

  - ❖ http://www.artauthority.net

- **Apps (applications):** Download to a device free or low-cost apps that offer engaging interactive activities and picture support for communication and learning new tasks. Many apps are listed in this chapter.

- **Email:** Use text to speech to read text aloud and voice recognition to enable the user to dictate messages to send as an email.

- **Texting:** Send messages to a cellphone or tablet from another cellphone or tablet.

- **Facebook.com (social networking site):** Send public or private messages to friends and family to stay in touch.

- **Internet browser:** Use Safari, Chrome, Mozilla Firefox, or other browsers on a tablet, smartphone, or computer to

  ❖ participate in an online social-networking site, such as Facebook, to view pictures of friends or stay in touch or re-establish contact with people;

  ❖ engage in a cognitively stimulating drill or task (http://www.lumosity. com);

  ❖ listen to a free college lecture (http://www.apple.com/education/ itunes-u).

Telephones

In addition to smartphones, there are special cell phones as well as landline phones that have helpful features for people with such challenges as cognitive deficits, hearing loss, visual impairments, limited dexterity, or difficulty speaking.

Cell phones ▨▨▨▨▨▨▨▨▨▨▨▨▨▨▨▨▨▨▨▨▨▨▨▨

When seniors are leaving their homes it is often very helpful if they get into the habit of carrying a cell phone, even if it is just for emergencies. Smartphones can be used in many helpful ways to help individuals with memory loss. Sophisticated phones can use GPS signals to track where the individual goes in case he or she becomes lost and confused. People with mild dementia can use cell phones to help them remember where they parked a car (pin the location using a map app), use GPS apps to help them find their way to desired locations, and have reminders embedded in a calendar app to help them stay on track.

Many smartphones are very complicated and have functionalities that may be overwhelming for seniors who are not computer savvy and who are used to using corded landline phones. There are special cell phones with only basic features that are most useful for older adults, such as those that have larger and more legible numbers and ones that can run health and medical apps for reminders to take or refill a medication or to access a registered nurse for health advice

- Jitterbug (http://www.greatcall.com/jitterbug)

- Samsung Galaxy (http://www.samsung.com/us/mobile)

- Doro PhoneEasy (http://www.doro.com)

Landline Phones

A corded telephone or landline is often the best choice for seniors experiencing memory loss because

- it is more familiar,

- it cannot be misplaced like a cell phone,

- it is typically simpler to use.

A wide range of landline phones are available that are very useful for older adults. Here are some great sites that feature these phones:

- Modern Senior Products (http://www.modernseniorproducts.com)

- 101Phones.com (http://www.101phones.com/cat/1928/Special-Needs-Home)

- OnlinePhoneStore.com (http://www.specialneeds.onlinephonestore.com)

eReaders

Many older individuals are initially reluctant to try using technology to read. The use of eReaders, however, has steadily increased since the first modern eReader became available in the late 1990s, and the devices are now used by a wide range of individuals, both young and old. Digital books, or ebooks, can be read on a desktop, laptop, tablet, smartphone, or dedicated device, such as an eReader. eReaders have become more affordable and offer many benefits for individuals with dementia, especially for those in the mild stages of the disease. Many of those in the more severe stages of dementia lose the joy of reading, and visually appealing interactive apps may be a more appropriate use of technology to continue to engage them.

For older adults, there are many benefits to reading from an eReader instead of a book, including the following:

- An eReader is usually lighter to hold than a book, so it can be used in a greater variety of reading positions and held by individuals with arthritic or weak hands.

- The font can easily be made larger.

- The eReader may have a text-to-speech option with high-quality voices. Listening to books read aloud as the user views the text offers the greatest comprehension and improves memory of the information. It is also ideal when the words are highlighted as they are read aloud. However, some publishers do not permit their books to be read aloud using the text-to-speech option.

- Books can be ordered from a library or online and downloaded directly to many eReaders. There is no need to go to a bookstore or library to get a book.

  ❖ Overdrive Media Console app, by OverDrive, Inc., is compatible with many devices and is used to download digital copies of books from the library (http://www.search.overdrive.com).

- Many books can fit onto one eReader.

- eReaders can be read with only one hand holding it and the other navigating between pages.

- There are many free ebooks available.

Quite a few eReaders are available, including the following:

- Nook from Barnes and Noble (http://www.barnesandnoble.com/NOOK)

- Kindle, by Amazon (http://www.amazon.com/kindle)

- Sony Reader (http://www.ebookstore.sony.com/reader)

- iPad Mini, by Apple (http://www.apple.com/ipad-mini)

Audiobooks

Many seniors enjoy listening to books read aloud by professionals. It is easier to remember a story when the individual reads the text aloud at the same time that he or she listens to the text being read aloud. Audiobooks also may be easier to understand than words said aloud by a computer using text to speech. Shorter stories are most appropriate for individuals who have a hard time remembering a complicated story line. To obtain an audiobook try one of the following:

- Search an online bookstore's selection of downloadable audiobooks, such as http://www.amazon.com or http://www.bn.com.

- Purchase an audio CD of a book.

- Visit an audiobook Web site, such as

  ❖ http://www.audible.com

- ❖ http://www.itunes.com

- ❖ http://www.simplyaudiobooks.com

- ❖ http://www.Librivox.com-0 (provides free public-domain narrated books)

Books as Apps

Some seniors may prefer "app books." A few examples include

- *You're Only Old Once!* (Dr. Seuss), by Oceanhouse Media. Offers interactive, engaging graphics and audio;

- 28,000 Funny Jokes, by Free Style (text only);

- Quotes Plus, by Decluttered Mind (text only).

Recording and Scanning Pens

There are quite a few specialized "pens" on the market that have video recorders, text to speech, or the ability to scan images. One pen, the Livescribe Pen, is especially helpful for individuals with memory challenges. The user writes on special paper after tapping an image on the paper to start the recording and everything is recorded as the person writes. Later, the person can tap on the paper and hear what was said at that time. A person does not have to be able to write to use the pen. Any physical mark will do. (More information can be found at http://www.livescribe.com.)

Here are a few other helpful uses of this type of pen:

- **Medical appointments:** An individual can ask a doctor to write in his or her special notebook using the Livescribe Pen while saying aloud the instructions for the person.

- **Activities of daily living:** Caregivers or practitioners can draw a picture, tape a photograph of an activity, or write the name of an activity on the special paper and then record step-by-step directions for a person with memory loss. They could write down the most important words and verbally provide additional explanations so that when the person touches the paper he or she can hear the words said aloud and recall the task or activity steps.

- **Photograph or memory book:** Family members and practitioners can create a personalized memory book using photographs mounted on the special paper, or attach some of the paper near a photograph in the book and print and record information about the picture.

Scanning pens are also very useful for individuals who want to save text or images. For example, the pen can be used to scan receipts, documents, or directions and then the images can be uploaded to a computer. An example of a scanning pen is the IRIS Pen (http://www.irislink.com), which instantly scans text, numbers, and images into any application and can then convert documents into editable text.

Selecting Apps, Software, and Web sites

When selecting apps, software, and Web sites, consider the following:

- The program should be easy to learn and use and should have clear instructions.

- For drill and practice apps, to limit frustration there should be a way to obtain help when the user is unable to independently complete a task.

- The text and images should be large, free from clutter, and visually appealing.

- It is helpful (but not critical) if scores can be saved and progress tracked.

- Content should be age appropriate and interesting. Many more technology tools are created for children than for adults with impaired cognition. Some adults are fine with using products created for children, while others may find them insulting.

- There should be an emphasis on visual supports for engagement and learning rather than a reliance on spoken narrative.

- It is helpful if the program can be customized to meet the needs of the user.

Searching for Appropriate Technology

The worlds of mainstream, educational, and assistive technologies are merging and rapidly evolving. More and more technologies are becoming available and affordable that have the potential of significantly improving the lives of people who have dementia and successfully engaging them in activities. The following are tips for choosing an appropriate technology for a person with dementia:

- Explore the Web sites of products listed in this chapter that appear to be the most appropriate in order to learn more about current features, pricing, and specifications. Search online for reviews and to learn about similar products. Many sites, such as iTunes, allow the user to view other apps or products purchased by other individuals who bought the item displayed.

- Search online via YouTube.com for videos of how to use a specific app or software product to help determine if it is a good fit.

- Take advantage of free trials and "lite" versions of apps prior to purchasing a product.

- Be creative. There is no one correct way to use a given product.

- Seek professional guidance from someone who is tech savvy and well versed in helping individuals with dementia.

- Subscribe to this author's free online newsletter at http://www.innovativespeech.com for a steady stream of helpful suggestions (typically twice a month) by entering your email in the upper right-hand corner.

- Check out the following blog sites, which primarily feature reviews of products for children, many of which are also appropriate for adults:

  ❖ http://www.bridgingapps.com: Bridging the gap between technology and people with disabilities

  ❖ http://www.iear.org: Educator reviews of educational apps

  ❖ http://www.commonsensemedia.org/guide/special-needs: Apps for individuals with special needs

Implementation Strategies

The following are tips for using technologies to assist someone with dementia:

- Start with what you already know. Many of us use technology, such as cell phones, smartphone cameras, email, texting, online maps, and networking sites in our daily routines, yet we do not think of ways to empower individuals with dementia to benefit from these tools. With simplified instructions and visual supports, many of the tools we take for granted can be used in stimulating activities for individuals with dementia.

- Follow the lead of the person you are helping. Watch for signs of engagement and interest. Keep activities enjoyable and personally relevant.

- Start simple. Provide all necessary help for initial success and then gradually withdraw support to promote learning.

Enhancing Strength-based Programming Using Technology

As discussed elsewhere in this book, each individual has multiple intelligences and it is most effective to offer tailored strength-based activities to promote enjoyment and success. The sections that follow are organized by each of the seven multiple intelligences and describe assistive technologies as well as interactive multisensory technologies that can be used in activities to engage people with dementia. This is not an all-inclusive list, but rather a sample of the types of technologies that are available both to stimulate the brain and compensate for weaknesses. Many of the items listed actually fall within the domain of more than one area of intelligence.

As mentioned earlier, the apps listed in this chapter generally refer to iOS apps that work on Apple products, such as the iPad. Many, however, are also available for use on other devices. Product features, pricing, and platforms—especially in this ever-changing technological world—continue to evolve, and, therefore, product Web sites are provided for reference.

At the time this chapter was written there were more than 830,000 active apps available through iTunes and over 650,000 active Android apps, an overwhelming number that continues to grow daily. It is difficult to search for apps that are appropriate for individuals with dementia. The listings in this chapter hopefully will assist you in researching and finding the appropriate apps and other technology tools.

Verbal-Linguistic

A wide range of products is available to assist those with verbal-linguistic strengths. The products listed below can be used to encourage and improve all forms of communication (speech, comprehension, reading, writing). Many of the products can be used to help individuals with dementia ranging from mild to more severe; the way they are used differs depending on the needs of the person. Some items can be used to improve verbal-linguistic tasks and others can be used when this is an area of weakness, to enhance functional communication skills. The Web sites, software products, and apps listed are intended to

- provide practice with communication and literacy skills and to compensate for difficulty speaking,

- make text easier to read online and improve reading comprehension by reading text aloud and providing tasks to improve reading comprehension,

- help individuals to write using voice and speech recognition technology.

Most of the products listed below are great for enhancing all aspects of language. The assistance of a speech-language pathologist is recommended to help evaluate the individual's speech and language strengths and weaknesses. Games on computers, tablets, and smartphones can neurologically stimulate many areas of the brain related to language and expression. Be sure to take advantage of the many accessibility features that tablets provide, including for the following scenarios for an individual who has dementia:

- If writing is easier than speaking, use text-to-speech features that read aloud what is written.

- If speaking is easier than writing, use the integrated microphone to have the device write out what is said aloud.

- If auditory is better than reading comprehension, enable the "speak selection" and "highlight accessibility" features to have the device read aloud whichever words you highlight or select on screen.

Web sites

- Language-based games
  - ❖ http://www.aarp.org/games
  - ❖ http://www.freerice.com
  - ❖ http://www.languagegames.org
  - ❖ http://www.sheppardsoftware.com
  - ❖ http://www.spellingcity.com
  - ❖ http://www.hasbro.com/scrabble/en_US/boggleGame.cfm
- Listen to a lecture
  - ❖ http://www.apple.com/education/itunes-u-
- Learn a new language
  - ❖ http://www.rosettastone.com
- Enhance the readability of web sites
  - ❖ http://www.readability.com
- Bring humor into language activities
  - ❖ http://www.riddlesandjokes.com
  - ❖ http://www.pmcaregivers.com/Humor.htm
  - ❖ http://www.pruneville.com/senior-jokes/
  - ❖ http://www.butlerwebs.com/jokes/default.htm

Computer software

- WordQ/SpeakQ, byGoQSoftware.com (http://www.goqsoftware.com). Software that offers voice recognition, word prediction, and text-to-speech support for computers.

- Reading Ally (http://www.readingally.org). This used to be called Recording for the Blind & Dyslexic. Compatible with computers and tablets.

- Natural Reader, by NaturalSoftware, Ltd. (http://www.Naturalreaders. com). Text-to-speech software for computers.

- Universal Reader Plus, by Premier Assistive (http://www. readingmadeez. com). Text-to-speech software and magnifier for computers.

Apps (for drill and practice)

- Dragon Dictation, by Nuance Communications. This voice recognition app requires no training and can be used to improve speech clarity by encouraging the user to "make the device understand what you say." It can also be used to compose messages for email, documents, or social networking sites.

- Grasshopperapps.com. Offers a wide array of very inexpensive customizable apps to improve many aspects of communication.

  ❖ Little Speller Sight Words

  ❖ Little Reader Four Letter Words

  ❖ Little Matchups

  ❖ Phototouch Concepts

- Lingraphica. A series of SmallTalk and TalkPath apps for adults who have language deficits.

  ❖ SmallTalk Conversational Phrases

  ❖ SmallTalk Daily Activities

  ❖ Lingraphica TalkPath Speaking

- Smarty Ears. Engaging interactive apps that are customizable and appropriate for adults. Note that the majority of the apps offered by this company are for children.

  ❖ Reading Rehabilitation Toolkit

  ❖ iName it

- Speak in Motion VAST. Especially helpful for individuals who have difficulty sequencing speech sounds and who benefit from viewing up-close mouth movement. These apps feature the simultaneous combination of visual, auditory, and, in some case, written cues.

- ❖ VAST tx: Key Words
- ❖ VAST tx: Therapy Samples

- Speech Sounds on Cue, by Multimedia Speech Pathology. An app that uses up-close mouth videos, photos, and sound clips with recording and playback as well as features to encourage independent practice of saying words grouped by initial speech sound.

- Tactus Therapy Solutions, by Tactus Therapy Solutions, Ltd. Apps produced by a speech pathologist who specializes in working with adults who have language challenges. Apps are customizable and intuitive.

- ❖ Language TherAppy
- ❖ Naming TherAppy
- ❖ Category TherAppy

- VocabularySpellingCity, by VocabularySpellingCity.com. An app with spelling and language games. The games are also offered via the company's web site.

Apps (for communication practice)

There are many apps that can be used to encourage conversation or as the focus of an activity to be discussed among a group of participants. They can also be used to create scenarios to help an individual practice expressing a need, offering feedback, and following as well as giving directions.

- My Playhome, by Shimon Young (http://www.myplayhomeapp.com)
- More Grillin', by Maverick Software (http://www.mavericksoftwaregames.com)
- Cookie Doodle, by Shoe the Goose (http://www.shoethegoose.com)
- Conversation Cards, by Wee Black Sheep Entertainment (http://www.weeblacksheep.com/apps/conversation-cards/)

Severely Impaired Communication Skills

As communication becomes more difficult, it becomes increasingly important to slow down the pace of the communication, support communication with visuals, reduce environmental distractions, and use nonverbal ways to communicate, such as touch, facial expression, and physical actions. Engage the individual in the present rather than quizzing him or her on the past or preparing for the future.

Picture-based Tools for Communication

Augmentative and Alternative Communication (AAC) can be used to assist those who have difficulty speaking and recalling words. There are a large number of devices, software products, and apps designed to help these individuals communicate. A comprehensive review of them is beyond the scope of this chapter. For more information, please refer to the following resources:

- AAC TechConnect (http://www.aactechconnect.com). Offers toolkits, online resources, and workshops that simplify the AAC evaluation process.

- United States Society for Augmentative and Alternative Communication, the national chapter of ISAAC, the International Society for Augmentative and Alternative Communication (http://www.ussaac.org)

- AAC-RERC (Rehabilitation Engineering Research Center, a collaborative research group dedicated to the development of effective AAC technology) (http://www.aac-rerc.psu.edu)

There are number of AAC apps that may be appropriate for individuals with dementia. As the severity of the dementia increases, so too does the need for the communicative partner to assume more of the burden of conversation and actively provide assistance to facilitate communication. The following apps are most effective when thoughtfully customized to meet the needs of the individual. Photographs and sometimes videos from a person's home or daily routine can be used to teach new tasks and facilitate communication.

- Communicaide: AAC/Speech Therapy, by ObjectGraph LLC. This AAC app was developed for adults and is customizable. All items are presented at once for the person to view. The user selects photos or phrases to communicate, including a body image with a pain meter.

- Proloquo2go, by AssistiveWare (http://www.proloquo2go.com). A full-featured AAC app that uses a combination of text and images with "dynamic display" (the ability to view more choices when an item is selected) with a variety of grid sizes.

- FreeSpeech, by Give Speech Foundation, Inc. A free AAC app that enables users to add photos and then group them into folders, as well as collaborate with others to share content.

- Speak Aid HD, by DeMentid Apps (http://www.dementidapps.blogspot.com). A low-cost AAC app with basic pictured messages accompanied by voice output ("I'm hot," "I'm cold," "I need my medication"), and a stick figure with a touch-to-speak feature that says the part of the body that is touched.

- Answers:YesNo HD, by Simplified Touch (http://www.simplifiedtouch. com/SimplifiedTouch/YesNoHD.html). A simple app that offers the ability to customize a two-choice response with an image, text, and sound. It is often especially helpful when an individual's yes/no response is inconsistent.

- AutisMate, by SpecialNeedsWare (http://www.autismate.com). A customizable communication and learning app that uses visual scene displays with the ability to integrate video.

Logical-Mathematical

Many software products and apps are available that appeal to individuals whose strengths relate to math, reasoning, logic, and problem solving as well as people who want to improve those types of skills. The Internet offers Web sites for brain fitness as well as for board and arcade games, many of which are free or inexpensive.

The products listed here can be used to encourage and improve tasks involving

- figuring out solutions to problems,

- sorting and categorizing information,

- working with mathematical problems,

- playing games,

- exploring patterns.

Web sites

- http://www.lumosity.com

- http://www.brainhq.positscience.com

- http://www.mybrainsolutions.com

- http://www.mybraintrainer.com

- http://www.brainready.com

- http://www.aarp.org/games

- http://www.playwithyourmind.com

- http://www.coolmath.com

- http://www.funbrain.com

- http://www.GCFLearnFree.org

Software

- http://www.dakim.com (An engaging brain fitness program for seniors.)

Apps

- Coin Math, by Recession Apps
- Watch That!, by Vratislav Kalenda
- Little Solver, by Grasshopperapps.com
- Basic Sequencing Skills, by Nth Fusion LLC
- Injini Child Development Game Suite, by NC Soft
- Jigsaw Box, by Sparkle Apps
- Spaced Retrieval TherAppy, by Tactus Therapy Solutions
- Things that Go Together, by Grasshopperapps.com
- Charge Your Brain HD, by Unusual Things
- Memory Matches 2, by IDC

Visual-Spatial

Many Web sites as well as apps are available and are ideal for individuals whose strength involves visual, spatial, and perceptual skills or who want to improve those skill areas. As with other areas of strength-based programming, many of the products can be used to help individuals who have from mild to more severe dementia; the way they are used differs depending on the needs of the person. The web sites, software products, and apps listed here can be used with people who show strengths in or who want to improve their ability in the following areas:

- drawing and coloring
- working with shapes and designs
- looking at pictures, videos, and shows
- visualizing concepts
- completing mazes and puzzles

Web sites

- Lumosity (http://www.Lumosity.com). A variety of cognitively stimulating tasks that reach very complex levels. Individuals using this site should have a relatively high tolerance for frustration. Closely tracks progress. App also available.

- Jigzone (http://www.jigzone.com). Users determine the pictures, number of pieces, and shape of each puzzle.

Software

- Dakim Brain Fitness, by Dakim, Inc. (http://www.dakim.com). Brain fitness software designed for adults over the age of 60. Uses positive encouragement through visually engaging videos, humor, and photography to stimulate six essential cognitive domains. Activities are appropriate for those with mild-to-moderate cognitive impairment.

Apps

- Injini: Child Development Game Suite, by NC soft. Simple puzzles and activities. Very clear and simple graphics and animations and small gradations between levels.

- Grasshopper apps, by GrasshopperApps.com. A wide variety of simple, customizable, and visually engaging apps, such as Tell Time, Count Money, Things that Go Together, and Sight Words.

- Tozzle, by Nodeflexion.com. Offers many puzzles of increasing difficulty with enticing graphics and sounds.

- Word Seek, by Idealiz, Inc. Word-search game.

- Visual Timer, by G. Van Geloven. A timer that slowly uncovers a photograph.

- PlayArt, by Tapook. Provides many canvases of famous masterpieces as well as videos about the artists. Encourages users to edit and create art.

- Ilovefireworks, by Fireworks Games. Touch the screen and watch fireworks appear.

- My Coloring Book and Free Paint, by Gortz Media. Simple, hand drawings to color and paint with bright colors.

- ArtStudio for iPad, by Lucky Clan. Draw, paint, and edit photographs.

- MatrixMatch, by MyFirstApp.com. Can be used to improve visual-perceptual skills.

- Visual Attention TherAppy, by Therapy Tactus Solutions, Ltd. Provides systematic visual scanning and cancellations tasks.

Tactile-Kinesthetic

Although tactile-kinesthetic tasks usually involve the manipulation of physical objects and physical activities, such as sports and exercise classes, there are technology tools and apps that appeal to those with this type of strength or that can be used to improve this area. The Web sites, software products, and apps listed here can enhance one's success with the following types of tasks:

- Engaging in movement, balance, and fitness activities

- Touching something (a button or screen) and seeing a resulting action

Game systems

- Nintendo Wii, by Nintendo (http://www.nintendo.com/wii). Playing a favorite sport, such as golf, bowling, tennis, dancing, or boxing, and engaging in general fitness and balance activities can be extremely beneficial for people with dementia by encouraging greater movement and socialization.

Web sites

- Exercise for Seniors (http://www.livestrong.com/senior-exercises). Offers a variety of videos that can be viewed online of exercises and exercise routines that are appropriate for seniors.

- Functional Skills Training (http://www.GCFLearnFree.org). Offers a variety of interactive activities to enhance functional skills (math, money).

Apps for Active Movement

Many apps are available that require active movement. As cognitive skills deteriorate, apps can be implemented with reduced cognitive demands. As with other apps, they can be made more or less difficult, depending on the expectations set up by the activity facilitator. They all offer visually engaging graphics and cause-and-effect relationships, and many are soothing.

- Cause and Effect Sensory Light Box, by Cognable. Encourages users to touch the screen to explore many scenes with high-quality audio and abstract visuals.

- Color Dots, by Ellie's Games. This app developer produces an array of apps for iOS (Apple) and Android devices that focus on basic eye–hand coordination, color recognition, and fine motor skills.

- Doodle Buddy, by Pinger, Inc. Offers a variety of writing tools, such as chalk, paint, or markers. Practice drawing pictures or writing letters or words. Play games, such as tic-tac-toe, on pre-made boards.

- Gavitarium 2, by Robert Neaugu. Blends music, art, and motion into a relaxing activity.

- Ilovefireworks, by Fireworks Games. Touch the screen and view a beautiful fireworks display.

- Make It Pop, by Tryangle Labs. A simple cause-and-effect app with activities such as rocket launching and popcorn, bubble, and balloon popping.

- My Coloring Book and Free Paint, by Gortz Media. Simple, hand drawings to color and paint with bright colors.

- Peekaboo Barn, by Night and Day Studios, Inc. Touch the screen to reveal an animal that is hiding. Encourages initiation of activity.

- Pocket Pond, by TriggerWave, LLC. This soothing game encourages the user to interact with beautiful ponds filled with aquatic life.

Auditory-Musical

Individuals with dementia can benefit from the relaxing or upbeat sounds of music. Memories of songs often provide a wonderful source of reminiscence, and people who may have difficulty speaking may be able to sing along to a song from their past or play along using an instrument. Individuals should be encouraged to actively interact with the music. It is often helpful to view large print lyrics while singing. The products listed here are available both for computers as well as mobile devices, and music is customized for needs of the listener.

- Free online customized music. Type a genre or the name of a song or artist to create and listen to a customized music station.

  ❖ http://www.Pandora.com

  ❖ http://www.iheartradio.com

- Music downloads. Songs can be purchased, downloaded, and played from computers or mobile devices.

  ❖ iTunes.com

  ❖ Google Music (music.google.com)

  ❖ Music CDs

  ❖ Sing Along with Eldersong (http://www.eldersong.com). CDs and large print lyrics.

  ❖ Video Respite (http://www.videorespite.com). Offers a series of CDs that are designed to hold the attention of people with dementia through music, light movement, and reminiscence.

- Apps

  ❖ Music Sparkles, by Kids Games Club. All-in-one musical instruments collection. Interactive music app encourages tapping and playing of many different instruments, such as a piano, xylophone, or guitar.

  ❖ Music Color, by SoundTouch. Listen to beautiful classical music and interact with colors and photographs.

  ❖ Fuji Leaves, by Andreas Ehnbom. An interactive music app. The individual uses leaves and falling stones to create music.

  ❖ VAST Songs, by SpeakinMotion. View and sing along to simple, repetitive songs by following close-up video of mouth movements combined with visual and auditory cues that allow individuals to readily produce speech.

  ❖ Music Healing/Voice, by XME. Soothing music and vocal performances to beautiful imagery that fade in and out.

Interpersonal

Individuals with interpersonal skills typically enjoy being with others and interacting with them during activities. Seniors are often quite isolated, but technology can alleviate the feeling of isolation. Many Web sites and apps are available that are ideal for individuals who benefit from increased social experiences. Most of the items listed below can be used to help those who have from mild to more severe dementia; the way they are used differs depending on the needs of the person. The Web sites, software products, and apps that appeal to those with interpersonal strengths can support or enhance the following areas:

- Communicating with others while seeing them

- Sharing experiences and interacting with others in person or online

As verbal communication and auditory comprehension deteriorate, it is very helpful to use nonverbal communication and to see people as you speak to them.

- Video calls. This feature is now integrated directly into a number of devices.

  ❖ http://www.google.com/talk

  ❖ http://www.google.com/hangouts

  ❖ http://www.skype.com

  ❖ FaceTime, by Apple (http://www.apple.com). Engage in video calls via an iPhone, iPad, or Mac desktop.

- Postcards (pictures and videos) (http://www.postcardsapp.com). Photos are sent from family and friends to someone automatically via a tablet. No interaction or technology experience is required to view the pictures and videos.

- Games can be played with others online:
  - ❖ Words with Friends, by Zynga (http://www.wordswithfriends.com)
  - ❖ Uno, by Gameloft
  - ❖ 4 in a Row, by EnsenaSoft

Intrapersonal

Individuals with intrapersonal preferences and strengths typically prefer to be by themselves or engage in activities on their own. They want to pursue their individual interests and focus on their experiences and accomplishments. The Web sites, software products, and apps listed below can improve the following intrapersonal skills:

- Writing and recording inner feelings and ideas
- Reflecting on self-interests and accomplishments
- Learning new skills privately

Web sites

- Create a personal profile on Facebook.com
- Edit family pictures and create family albums on sites such as http://www. snapfish.com or http://www.shutterfly.com
- Learn the basics of a new language at http://www.busuu.com or http:// www.livemocha.com
- Document and research genealogy using tools, such as http://www. Ancestry.com

Software

- Microsoft PowerPoint and Microsoft Word (or other word processing program). Create a life story using pictures and text.

Apps

- Pictello, by AssistiveWare. Create a talking photo album.
- ArtStudio, by Lucky Clan for the iPad. Draw, paint, and edit photographs.
- My Daily Journal, by Jl Software Company, LLC. A simple, full-featured journal.

- iPhoto, by Apple. Edit pictures and videos.

- Ancestry, by Ancestry.com. Build, update, and share family tree.

- My Coloring Book, by Gortz Media. Simple, hand drawings to color and paint with bright colors.

Naturalistic ▨▨▨▨▨▨▨▨▨▨▨▨▨▨▨

Individuals with naturalistic preferences and strengths tend to be interested in being outdoors or learning about the environment and nature. Below are Web sites, software products, and apps for individuals who have strengths and interests in nature.

Web sites

- National Geographic (http://www.kids.nationalgeographic.com) has beautiful graphics, games, puzzles, and interactive activities.

- Discovery Channel (http://www.dsc.discovery.com)

- The Weather Channel (http://www.weather.com)

Apps

- Star Walk for iPad, by Vito Technology, Inc. Interactive astronomy guide

- National Geographic apps, by National Geographic Society. Offers a variety of apps, including

  ❖ *National Geographic* magazine

  ❖ National Parks

  ❖ National Geographic World Atlas

  ❖ National Geographic Today (takes you on a simulated trip around the world)

- Magic Window Living Pictures, by Jetson Creative, LLC. Beautiful, soothing, time-lapsed scenes with relaxing soundtracks.

- Music Healing, by XME-Relaxing. Music with beautiful nature graphics.

- WeatherBug, by Earth Networks. Offers real-time weather forecasts, alerts, and more.

- iDress for Weather, by Pebro Productions. Provides visual assistance using GPS technology and customizable closets.

- Kids Can Match, by Kids Place. Interactive adaptive memory game.

Tailor Activities for Each Individual

There is no exact right or wrong way to use a specific tool of technology to create "the perfect" activity for an individual who has dementia. Clinicians, caregivers, and family members need to keep an open mind, think about the strengths of the individual, and tap into those areas when creating an activity in order to maximize success and enjoyment.

It is usually preferable to start with technologies that the facilitator is already familiar with using. For instance, using pictures taken by a cell phone or iPad can be the basis for very enjoyable activities for individuals with varied remaining competencies. If a person is able to learn to take pictures with a smartphone or tablet, it is often enlightening to observe which kinds of pictures he or she takes to learn more about what the person is interested in and to use that insight to create activities based on those areas of interest. In addition to taking pictures, there are many ways photographs can be used in activities for seniors who have different areas of strengths.

Verbal-Linguistic

- Name the people and items in the photos.

- Speak in phrases and sentences about the photos.

- Label the photos with text and audio using apps, such as

    ❖ Phonto, by youthhr. A simple application that allows you to add text to pictures.

    ❖ Click n' Talk, by Intermediate District 287. Import photos or Web images, create a text presentation, and record a message.

    ❖ Tapikeo, by Jean-Eudes Lepelletier. Easily and quickly create audio-enabled picture books.

Intrapersonal

- Reflect on and recall personal experiences that were captured in images.

- Create a journal using apps, such as

    ❖ My Wonderful Days, by haha Interactive

    ❖ iDiary for Kids, by Tipitap, Inc. Journaling platform for writing and drawing

    ❖ Speech Journal, by Mobile Education Store

    ❖ Pictello, by AssistiveWare

Visual-Spatial

- Spend time editing and viewing pictures, recalling people and places, adding special effects to photos and creating collages.

  - ❖ Snapseed, by Nik Software, Inc.

  - ❖ Photo Collage HD Pro, by chen kaiqian

  - ❖ Pic Collage, by Cardinal Blue

Interpersonal

- Take pictures of family and friends (still and video).

- Share pictures with others by sending them online via email or posting them for family to see (Facebook.com; Flikr.com; Shutterfly.com).

Logical-Mathematical

- Organize photographs and label them using apps, such as

  - ❖ Photo Manager Pro, by Linkus

  - ❖ Pics, by Phyar Studio

  - ❖ Photo Sort, by Romain Henry

Naturalistic

- Take and view pictures of plants, animals, the sky, and other settings from nature.

Auditory-Musical

- View video clips of musical performances and conversations.

- Add audio to pictures using apps, such as

  - ❖ Pictello, by AssistiveWare

  - ❖ Fotobabble (http://www.fotobabble.com)

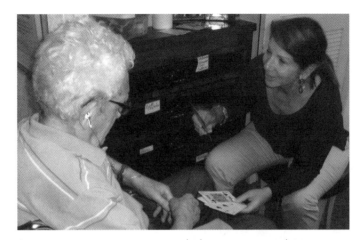

A caregiver engaging a person with dementia in a card game

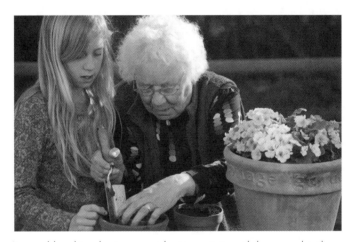

A granddaughter sharing a gardening activity with her grandmother

Chapter 6

Practical Tips for Enhancing Communication with Adults with Dementia

Communication, a key aspect in human relations, is the connection between individuals. Maintaining an individual's ability to communicate preserves his or her quality of life. For a practitioner or caregiver to engage an individual with a neurodegenerative disease in conversation means assuming the role of conversational leader, or one who initiates all discussions and structures statements and questions in a fashion that prompts responses. Most older adults who have Alzheimer's disease and other dementias still desire to communicate, but they are unable to initiate conversations. Being responsible for maintaining the flow of conversation involves leading, prompting, and guiding these individuals to engage in conversation. Structuring conversations is similar to leading another individual in an unfamiliar dance. Unaware of the actual dance steps, the person is unable to participate alone; by following the steps and motions of a lead dancer, however, he or she moves successfully and appropriately to the music. Likewise, an adult with Alzheimer's disease can successfully engage in verbal interactions when he or she has a conversation leader who initiates and maintains the flow of the dialogue or the "conversational dance." The adult with moderate to severe dementia may lack communication skills, but still has the capacity to enjoy the process of conversing as well as the social acceptance and recognition gained from relating to another person. Danielle N. Ripich's books, *Alzheimer's Disease Communication Guide: The FOCUSED Program for Caregivers* (1996 and 2005 revised edition), are excellent resources for both caregivers and elder care practitioners for communication techniques to maintain verbal interactions with adults who have Alzheimer's disease.

Using a strength-based approach enables speech–language pathologists, activity therapists, caregivers, nursing staff, and family members to select personally meaningful topics or visual cues related to an individual's remaining strengths and preferences to prompt communication. For example, if an individual displays visual and naturalistic preferences, pictures of animals and plants are meaningful conversation topics. Animal picture books, magazines, and cards would spark recall and engage the older adult in conversations.

Using a strength-based approach also enables practitioners to know *what* to say to an individual who has dementia, which is the first step in creating successful communications. The next step involves knowing *how* to speak to an individual who possesses waning conversation skills, which the next section addresses.

Communication Techniques

Basic developmental language strategies, such as modeling responses, elaborating details, and repetition and expansion of utterances, as well as speaking in short, simple sentences, assist a conversation leader in structuring meaningful discussions with an older adult with Alzheimer's disease. It is useful to eliminate all professional jargon when speaking to the individual, as well as to his or her family members, and instead use simple, everyday language to provide straightforward directions. Constant reinforcement of communication and strength-based strategies in a patient's daily routine and environment will enable the person to communicate for as long as possible.

Written guides that include tips to reinforce a practitioner's verbal recommendations can be used to facilitate clear-cut communications among professional staff members and improve communications between staff and family members. The guides are also useful resources for family members and personal caregivers if the individual with dementia resides at home. Family members, for example, who are experiencing the emotional throes of a relative's behavioral outbursts and communication problems usually become overwhelmed with an abundance of medical and therapeutic information. Precise written instructions, such as those in the Memory Loss Caregiver Guide, enhance family members' awareness of a relative's strengths and limitations as well as what to say to their loved one. Both professionals and family members should be on the same page when it comes to knowing what to say to a person whose ability to communicate is compromised by Alzheimer's disease.

The following groups of tips offer practical, straightforward suggestions for how family members and healthcare practitioners can improve conversations and interactions with individuals who have dementia. Geriatric care professionals, for example, can use these recommendations to enhance family consultations, staff and caregiver training sessions, and support group meetings. To assist the individuals with Alzheimer's to verbalize for as long as possible, it is important for family members and professionals to use the same strategies and to use them consistently. All suggestions in this section are useful for family members and caregivers who are working with an individual at home and for practitioners working with people who have dementia who are living in a long-term care or assisted living facility. It is the author's hope that employing these techniques will create moments of joy for both the person with dementia as well as his or her conversation leader or partner.

Helping Children to Communicate with an Older Relative Who Has Dementia

Alzheimer's disease affects all family members, including children. An individual may live as long as 20 years with the effects of the disease. This "long good-bye" may span a youngster's entire childhood, from birth through adolescence or even into adulthood, and may deprive a child of pleasant memories of an older relative. Children are more apt to cope with an older relative's dementia when they understand the nature of their relative's disease. For example, a parent or other adult family member can read an age-appropriate book about Alzheimer's to a child or encourage an older child to read books about Alzheimer's disease. (Appendix C lists recommended readings on Alzheimer's disease for children.) Talk to a child about an older relative's life story and current illness. Once a child understands better why an elder has cognitive and memory difficulties, create opportunities for him or her to relate to this family member. For example, encourage the child to bring puzzles and wooden blocks to share with the relative. Many elders with dementia respond to these simple tactile-kinesthetic activities.

Visiting a relative with dementia who resides in an assisted living memory unit or long-term care facility requires preparation. Instead of sitting idly by and observing the slow deterioration of a loved one, family members should plan activities that improve a visit. One preparation involves a show-and-tell activity in which family members bring items to share with their relative. These shared items become the focal point of each visit. A child can be encouraged to contribute to show-and-tells by being given an opportunity to make something for the relative. Planned visits and structured conversations enable a family to interact with their loved one for as long as possible.

Creating Meaningful and Enjoyable Visits with a Relative Who Has Dementia

Visiting an adult with dementia at times can be stressful for the individual as well as for the visitor. This is true whether the person resides at home or in an assisted living facility, special memory care unit, or long-term care facility. The two lists of tips that follow can be used by family members to engage meaningfully with a loved one during a visit while also easing the stress and challenges in communicating with the individual. Adena Joltin, author of *A Different Visit: Activities for Caregivers and Their Loved ones with Memory Impairments* (2005), notes that meaningful and engaging visits are an important part of daily life for a relative with memory impairment, wherever he or she lives. "If they cannot remember the details of the visit," Joltin writes, "it is not really important. The positive feelings they have because of a good visit can linger afterward, for them and for you. Activities serve a much greater function than just making it easier to have a visit. They allow us to rediscover the person who is hidden by the deficits." (2005, p. ii)

Tips to Enrich Conversations with a Person with Alzheimer's Disease or a Related Dementia

- Look directly at the person when you speak.

- Introduce yourself before starting a conversation. State your name!

- Address the individual using the correct title or preferred name. For example, say, "Hi, Dad. It's Tom," or "Hi, Aunt Sally! It's your niece, Josephine," or "Hello, Mrs. Jones! It's Mary, your aide."

- Initiate conversations by introducing the topic. Do not wait for the individual to start talking. For example, "Let's look at the photos of your new greatgrandson."

- Smile. Speak in a loving manner.

- Offer only one idea at a time.

- Use simple words and short sentences.

- Speak slowly and clearly.

- Use gestures to accentuate your speech.

- Ask simple yes or no questions instead of open-ended questions. For example, ask, "Would you like a pudding?" Do not ask, "What do you want to eat?"

- Use multiple-choice questions instead of open-ended questions. For example, ask, "Would you like tea or coffee?" Do not ask, "What do you want to drink?"

- When repeating a question, use the same words.

- Introduce new people or new topics by providing the individual with an introduction. For example, say, "Mike is coming to see you today. Mike is your brother. Last time you played cards with Mike. Today, Mike is going to play another game of cards with you."

- Arrange opportunities for the individual to speak to children and to interact with pets, which encourage the person to use automatic expressions, such as "You're a good dog," "Give me your paw," "Sit down," and "Come."

- Use picture cards and picture books as conversation topics.

- When needed, use written questions and statements to help the person understand what you are saying.

Engaging and Communicating with People Who Have Dementia: Finding and Using Their Strengths, by Eileen Eisner.
Copyright © 2013, by Health Professions Press, Inc.

Tips to Encourage Communication with a Person with Severe Cognitive, Memory, and Communication Losses

- Use a personalized memory book, scrapbook, or wallet of photographs of significant people and events in the person's life as conversation topics and to prompt recall and short conversations about the individual's early life.

- Use a gentle touch to gain attention.

- Allow individuals additional time to formulate their thoughts into words.

- Maintain excellent eye contact. Look directly at the individual.

- Speak in short phrases and sentences.

- Use objects and pictures to demonstrate what you are saying.

- Label all displayed or framed photographs in the individual's living quarters. Engage the person in conversations about his or her important loved ones.

- Use a memory box of treasured objects to prompt recall.

- When possible, use pictures to initiate conversations.

- Play familiar songs and other music to encourage a sing-a-long.

- Play family CDs of familiar and significant events, such as weddings, picnics, or birthdays, to prompt recall.

- Allow the individual to hold and speak to plush toys or baby dolls that were designed especially for adults with cognitive and memory loss.

- Play the person's favorite music to spark attention and recall.

- Recognize and verbalize any communication responses in the forms of eye contact, facial expressions, and hand gestures. For example, say, "Mary, I know by the way you're smiling that you like what I said."

- Create situations for the individual to use automatic social expressions, such as "Thanks a lot," "See you later," and "Hi, how are you?"

Tips for What to Avoid When Speaking with a Person with Dementia

- Don't address the individual as a child. Speak in an adult manner.

- Don't yell. The loud volume and angry facial expression will only agitate and confuse the person.

- Don't interrupt the individual while he or she is speaking. Give the person opportunities to complete his or her thoughts.

- Don't talk about the individual in his or her presence as if he or she isn't there. Respect the person's dignity.

- Don't question the individual about recent events, which may not be recalled.

- Don't ask lengthy, complex questions, such as "Do you know who's coming to visit you on Sunday?"

- Don't ask questions that require the individual to recall names.

- Don't speak to the individual when he or she is not facing you. Face the individual when speaking directly to him or her.

- Don't engage a person in communications when the environment is filled with distracting noises, music, or activities.

- Don't try to reason or explain *why* to the individual. Use simple words and a reassuring tone when coaxing the person to do something.

- Don't argue. Instead, change the subject.

- Don't force the individual to do something. Instead, change the environment or change the subject.

- Don't wait for the person to speak. Initiate all conversations.

- Don't tell lengthy stories without the aid of pictures.

- Don't whisper.

- Don't speak too quickly.

- Don't pressure the individual to speak. Accept listening and maintaining eye contact as acceptable forms of connecting.

- Don't demand words as a response. Accept facial expressions, eye contact, and hand gestures as communication.

- Don't quiz the individual.

Engaging and Communicating with People Who Have Dementia: Finding and Using Their Strengths, by Eileen Eisner. Copyright © 2013, by Health Professions Press, Inc.

- Don't expect lengthy conversations. Engaging individuals in brief conversations is sufficient.

- Don't discuss two or more ideas at one time. Focus on one topic.

- Don't give a memory test by asking questions such as "Who am I?" or "What's my name?"

- Don't give up!

Tips to Promote Successful Interactions between Children and a Relative with Dementia

- Encourage children to bring plush teddy bears and other stuffed animals. Many adults with dementia enjoy touching the fuzzy fabrics and ribbons. Some relatives might respond to life-like baby dolls by speaking or singing to them.

- Label all framed photographs in an individual's living quarters, including old, familiar family photos. Encourage children to ask their relative about these photographs each time they come to visit.

- When possible, have children play simple games with their relative, such as Candy Land, picture bingo, and lotto.

- Gather some of the individual's personal objects and souvenirs (e.g., change purse, costume jewelry, keys, library card, makeup case, commemorative pins and badges) in a memory box that can be used to initiate enjoyable discussions between a child and a relative with dementia. Encourage the relative to touch the items. The tactile-kinesthetic sensation of handling these meaningful objects may prompt reminiscences and stimulate conversations.

- Encourage children to sing and perform familiar songs for their older relative. Surprisingly, people with dementia may be able to recite all the words to their favorite old songs, but are not able to engage in meaningful conversations. Singing with older relatives will produce shared family interactions. In some cases, older adults who do not sing will be able to participate by smiling and moving to the music.

- Have a child bring familiar nursery rhymes and storybooks, such as the *The Three Bears,* to read with their relative. Don't be surprised if the relative begins to recite these rhymes along with the child.

- Use familiar magazines with pictures, such as *National Geographic,* to engage the individual with dementia in conversation. Encourage children to look at the pictures and turn the pages for their relative. Garage sales are wonderful places to find vintage magazines and old books, such as the Dick and Jane readers.

- Watch familiar movies, such as *Hello Dolly,* together and reminisce about the movie stars and the movie itself.

- Play CDs of familiar television shows, such as *The Jack Benny Show* and *The Ed Sullivan Show,* to prompt reminiscence about how things used to be back then.

- Use family photo albums as conversation starters between the generations.

Engaging and Communicating with People Who Have Dementia: Finding and Using Their Strengths, by Eileen Eisner. Copyright © 2013, by Health Professions Press, Inc.

- Do a family scrapbooking activity in which each time children visit their loved one they all work together to create a new page for the book. This shared activity involves cutting, pasting, and organizing photographs, pictures, and mementos that would encourage recall and prompt conversations. Also, children can look back at previous scrapbook pages with their relative prior to starting a new page together. It becomes a wonderful routine that gives children a sense of real purpose for their visits. How nice it is to hear a child say, "Let's visit grandpa, because we need to work on his scrapbook."

- When there is not much to say and little to show, reminisce about family history. Play familiar family CDs, movies, or videos of special occasions, such as weddings, picnics, and birthday parties. Family movies from the past show children the way things used to be while also encouraging a relative with memory loss to recall events.

- When the weather permits, invite the relative to come outside for a while. Encourage the individual to talk about what he or she sees and hears. Let the relative watch visiting children run and play outside the confines of a residential setting.

- Bring snack foods for children to share with their relative. Certain familiar foods, such as a Dixie cup of ice cream, might spark recall and encourage conversations between a child and his or her relative as they share a pleasant activity.

- Children might want to bring coloring books and/or puzzle books to share with their loved one.

Tips to Assist Family Members in Communicating with a Relative Who Has Alzheimer's Disease or a Related Dementia

- Use family photographs to create a personalized memory book of the individual's life. Use the photographs in the memory book to encourage a relative to talk about his or her childhood and early life. Bear in mind that recalling events from long-term memory is easier than recalling recent events. A simple, uncluttered book of family pictures enables adults with memory loss to reminisce about their personal experiences. For information on how to create a memory book, refer to *Memory and Communication Aids for People with Dementia,* by Michelle Bourgeois.

- Decorate the person's room with meaningful and familiar artwork or posters that relate to the individual's previous interests and hobbies. Point to the wall art to use the pieces as conversation starters.

- Create a visitor sign-in chart and display it in the individual's room. This will help a relative during the early phase of the disease to recall visits and to avoid asking, "Why don't you come to visit me?" During each visit, write a brief description on the sign-in chart, for instance: "December 14, 2013: It was your 95th birthday and we had a family party. We sang "Happy Birthday" and gave you a birthday cake with your picture on it. All your children, grandchildren, and great-grandchildren were here. Everyone helped you blow out all of the birthday candles. It was a wonderful visit. Love, Paula, Sam, and Evan."

- Gather some of the individual's personal objects, such as keys, old wallet, photographs, pens, paperweights, and so forth, in a small storage box. Use this memory box to initiate enjoyable discussions. Encourage the individual to touch the items. The tactile-kinesthetic sensation of handling these meaningful objects may prompt reminiscence.

- Play CDs of songs from familiar movies. Nostalgia plays an important role in enabling an individual to converse in a meaningful manner. The person's memory of events from long ago is keener than that of current events.

- Engage a relative in sing-alongs. Surprisingly, a person with dementia may be able to recite all the words to a favorite song but cannot engage in meaningful conversations. Singing is an enjoyable activity. In some cases, the older adult may show pleasure by smiling and moving to the music.

- Use familiar magazines, such as *Newsweek, Reader's Digest, People,* and *National Geographic,* to engage a relative in conversation.

- Reminisce about family history. Play old family movies to stimulate the relative's long-term memory. Use photo books from past weddings and special events to share with your loved one.

- When the weather permits, invite the relative to go for a walk. Once outside, engage him or her in conversation by commenting on the surroundings, such as the trees, cars, clouds, and flowers.

- When permitted, bring small pets or babies with you. Dogs, cats, and babies usually prompt the individual to utter automatic expressions, such as "What a cute baby! How old is she?" or "What's his name?," as well as traditional rhymes, such as "Patty Cake."

- Show the individual large-picture commercial brochures, such as car and travel brochures, to stimulate conversations.

- Providing the individual with a manicure and/or hand massage is a pleasant, shared activity.

Engaging and Communicating with People Who Have Dementia: Finding and Using Their Strengths, by Eileen Eisner.
Copyright © 2013, by Health Professions Press, Inc.

Tips for Professional Caregivers in Communicating with Individuals Who Have Moderate to Severe Dementia

- Never take the patient by surprise. Greet him or her directly from the front.

- Always address the individual by his or her preferred name. Some individuals do not respond to their first names or nicknames. Check to see if the person responds to a more formal form of address, such as Mr. Johnson.

- Introduce yourself before speaking. Even if you think the person knows you, say your name before asking a question or making a request.

- Look at the person's face when you speak.

- Start all conversations by introducing the topic. Tell the person what you're going to do before doing it. As you're doing something, describe exactly what you're doing. For example, say, "I'm combing your hair."

- Smile and speak in a calm manner.

- Offer only one suggestion at a time.

- Use single words, short phrases, and simple sentences.

- Give the individual time to respond to your statements and questions.

- Speak in a conversational tone and pitch. Do not shout or whisper.

- Ask multiple-choice questions, such as "Would you like to go to the solarium or the TV room?"

- Ask questions that require a yes or no response, such as "Are you cold?" Do not ask, "How's the temperature in here?"

- Do not interrupt what an individual is saying when he or she is trying to speak. Give the person an opportunity to complete his or her thoughts.

- Do not speak to an adult as if he or she is a child. Speak in an accepting, mature manner.

- When repeating questions, use the same words. Do not paraphrase or change your words.

- Encourage the person to reminisce. Old memories are more invigorating than recent events.

- If the individual has good visual acuity, provide written and visual cues as reminders. Do not rely entirely on verbal cues.

Engaging and Communicating with People Who Have Dementia: Finding and Using Their Strengths, by Eileen Eisner. Copyright © 2013, by Health Professions Press, Inc.

- Use memory books, memory boxes, and family videos to encourage communication.

- When all else fails, and if the person's vision is adequate, try to use communication picture boards to assist the person in expressing his or her needs.

- Eye contact and gestures are forms of communication. Accept any form of communication to engage an individual in the experience of connecting with another person.

Identifying the Behaviors of Individuals with Cognitive Impairment

These lists of recognizable behaviors is categorized according to each intelligence and further classified from higher- to lower-functioning skills to coordinate with the mild, moderate, and severe phases of a progressive dementia.

Verbal-Linguistic

Spoken Language

- Responds to jokes and humor

- Reminisces

- Speaks in sentences

- Talks to others

- Responds to verbal instructions

- Speaks to small children and pets

- Uses automatic social expressions, such as "How are you?" and "Good morning"

- Attempts to verbalize

- Responds to words

- Uses eye contact and gestures to communicate with others

Visual Language

- Reads

- Appears to read magazines

- Responds to the visual arts (movies, graphics, paintings)
- Responds to signs and posters
- Responds to picture cues
- Recognizes and describes pictures

Written Language

- Writes at length
- Reads and writes notes and letters
- Uses writing to communicate
- Prints words
- Draws shapes, letters, and numbers
- Uses pencil in an attempt to write
- Uses markers, chalk, or crayons to make letters, lines, or circular shapes

Logical-Mathematical

- Engages in computer activities
- Finds reasons for events
- Needs to know the rules
- Needs to know the time
- Does simple math calculations
- Plays simple board games and card games
- Performs best with order and reason
- Responds to time schedules
- Attempts to complete puzzles
- Organizes objects (sorts and classifies)
- Recognizes patterns and shapes

Visual-Spatial

Visual

- Responds to the visual arts (graphics, sculpture)
- Notices interior decorations
- Notices color, line, and texture

- Responds to visual aids and signs
- Responds to visual cues
- Responds to pictures and photos
- Watches TV and videos

Visual-Motor

- Writes, draws, and illustrates
- Draws simple pictures
- Doodles and draws abstract designs
- Sews or constructs models (cars, planes, boats)
- Uses clay, paint, and other media
- Uses yarn, fabrics, and other media

Tactile-Kinesthetic

- Participates in sports (golf, tennis, bowling)
- Dances, exercises, and marches to music
- Responds to relaxation exercises
- Enjoys walking
- Uses hand gestures to express ideas
- Enjoys moving around
- Often taps feet or fingers
- Responds to physical therapy
- Uses movement to express thoughts
- Uses hands to fix things
- Builds, sews, knits, and cuts
- Responds to arts and crafts
- Enjoys touching objects
- Enjoys touching textures
- Responds to recreational therapy
- Responds to massage therapy
- Responds to touch

Auditory-Musical

- Recognizes different languages
- Speaks two or more languages
- Rhymes words
- Recites jingles, rhymes, or poems
- Listens to music
- Responds to music therapy
- Listens to the radio
- Relaxes to music
- Hums songs
- Sings words to songs
- Plays a musical instrument
- Dances and moves to music
- Taps feet or claps hands to music
- Responds to a speaker's vocal tone
- Responds to vocal pitch and volume

Interpersonal

- Participates in group activities
- Responds to support groups
- Seeks company of others
- Participates in social events
- Sympathetic to others' feelings
- Responds to collaborative projects
- Offers assistance to others
- Likes to give advice
- Responds positively to visitors
- Sensitive to another's eye contact and body language
- Generally cooperates and shares
- Seeks new friends

- Uses social interactions to relax
- Uses social and polite expressions
- Enjoys watching others perform
- Is comforted by the company of others

Intrapersonal

- Responds to individual counseling
- Works alone at own pace
- Produces creative and original work
- Expresses individuality
- Is intuitive and perceptive
- Maintains a sense of self-esteem
- Expresses personal feelings
- At times aware of cognitive loss
- Relaxes alone
- At times needs reassurance
- Vulnerable sense of self-worth
- Needs to feel important
- Needs to be noticed by others

Naturalistic

- Enjoys outdoor walks and excursions (parks, zoos)
- Likes to garden
- Exhibits understanding of and interest in the natural sciences
- Enjoys indoor plant care
- Responds to and enjoys domestic pets
- Enjoys interacting with nature (e.g., watching birds, insects, and animals)
- Aware of seasonal changes and daily weather
- Responds to pictures of outdoor scenes, plants, flowers, and animals
- Responds to TV and videos of natural scenery and animals

- Responds and relaxes to audiotapes of nature sounds (i.e., rain, ocean, wind)
- Shows interest in the outdoors
- Enjoys sitting in sunlight
- Enjoys sitting in a solarium
- Seems less agitated when by a window

Recommended Readings for Family Members, Caregivers and Professionals

Bayles, K., & Tomoeda, C. (1993). *The ABCs of dementia*. Tucson, AZ: Canyonlands.

Bell, V. (2008). *The Best Friends book of Alzheimer's activities (volume two)*. Baltimore: Health Professions Press.

Bell, V. (2004). *The Best Friends book of Alzheimer's activities (volume one)*. Baltimore: Health Professions Press.

Bell, V. (2003). *The Best Friends approach to Alzheimer's care*. Baltimore: Health Professions Press.

Bell, V. (2001). *The Best Friends staff: Building a culture of care in Alzheimer's programs*. Baltimore, MD: Health Professions Press.

Bourgeois, M. S. (2007). *Memory books and other graphic cuing systems: Practical communication and memory aids for adults with dementia*. Baltimore: Health Professions Press.

Bourgeois, M. S., & Hickey, E. (2009). *Dementia: From diagnosis to management—A functional approach*. New York: Psychology Press.

Bowlby, C. (1993). *Therapeutic activities with persons disabled by Alzheimer's disease and related disorders*. Gaithersburg, MD: Aspen Press.

Brackey, J. A. (2007). *Creating moments of joy for the person with Alzheimer's or dementia (4th edition)*. Indiana: Purdue University Press.

Brawley, E. C. (1997). *Designing for Alzheimer's disease: Strategies for creating better care environments*. New York: John Wiley & Sons.

Buettner, L., & Martin, S. L. (1995). *Therapeutic recreation in the nursing home*. State College, PA: Venture.

Callone, P., Vasiloff, B., Brumback, R., Maternach, J., & Kudlacek, A. (2006). *A Caregiver's guide to Alzheimer's disease: 300 tips for making life easier*. New York: Demos Medical Publishing.

Coste, J. K. (2003). *Learning to speak Alzheimer's*. London: Vermilion.

de Klerk-Rubin, V. (2008). *Validation techniques for dementia care: The family guide to improving communication*. Baltimore: Health Professions Press.

Feil, N., & de Klerk-Rubin, V. (2012). *The Validation Breakthrough (3rd edition)*. Baltimore: Health Professions Press.

Genova, L. (2009). *Still Alice*. New York: Gallery Books.

Joltin, A., Camp, C. J., Noble, B. H., & Antenucci, V. M. (2005). *A different visit: Activities for caregivers and their loved ones with memory impairments*. Ohio: Myers Research Center.

Kindig, M.N., & Carnes, C. (1993). *Coping with Alzheimer's disease and other dementing illnesses*. San Diego, CA: Singular Publishing Group.

Larkin, M. (1995). *When someone you love has Alzheimer's*. New York: Dell.

Lazear, D. (1994). *Multiple intelligence approaches to assessment: Solving the assessment conundrum*. Tucson, AZ: Zephyr Press.

Mace, N. L., & Rabins, P. V. (2011). *The 36-hour Day: A family guide for caring for people who have Alzheimer's disease, related dementias, and memory loss (5th edition)*. Baltimore: The Johns Hopkins University Press.

McCone, V. (2003). *Butterscotch sundaes: My mom's story of Alzheimer's*. Sanborn, MN: Autumn Sparrow Press.

Moffett, P. (2007). *Ice cream in the cupboard*. Great Neck, NY: Garrison-Savanna Publishing, LLC.

Powell, L. S., & Courtice, K. (1993). *Alzheimer's disease: A guide for families*. Reading, MA: Addison-Wesley.

Rau, M. T. (1993). *Coping with communication challenges in Alzheimer's disease*. San Diego, CA: Singular Publishing Group.

Reisberg, B. (1988). Functional assessment staging (FAST). *Psychopharmacology Bulletin, 24*, 653–659.

Reisberg, B., Ferris, S. H., de Leon, M. J., & Crook, T. (1982) The global deterioration scale for assessment of primary degenerative dementia. *American Journal of Psychiatry, 139*, 1136–1139.

Ripich, D. (2005) Revised FOCUSED Caregiver's Guide: Communicating with persons with Alzheimer's Disease. The FOCUSED program for Caregivers. Insight Media.

Sheridan, C. (1995). *Failure-free activities for the Alzheimer's patient*. New York: Dell.

Silvermarie, S. (1996). *Tales from my teachers on the Alzheimer's unit*. Milwaukee, WI: Families International.

Simpson, C. (1996). *At the heart of Alzheimer's*. Gaithersburg, MD: Manor Healthcare.

Sparks, N. (1996). *The notebook*. New York: Warner Books.

Wexler, N. (1996). *Mama can't remember anymore*. Thousand Oaks, CA: Wein & Wein.

Wilkens, D. K. (1996). *Multiple intelligences activities*. Huntington Beach, CA: Teacher Created Materials.

Ziegler, R. C. (2009). *Let's look together: An interactive picture book for people with Alzheimer's and other forms of memory loss*. Baltimore: Health Professions Press.

Recommended Readings about Alzheimer's Disease for Children and Adolescents

■■■■■ ■■■■■■ ■■■■ ■■■■ ■■■■ ■■■ ■■■■■■ ■■■ ■■■

For additional, updated resources for children, go to the Alzheimer's Association Web site (http://www.alz.org). See the section titled Just for Kids & Teens.

Acheson, A. (2009). Grandpa's music: A story about Alzheimer's. Morton Grove, IL: Albert Whitman & Co.

American Health Assistance Foundation. (1997). *Fading memories: An adolescent's guide to Alzheimer's disease*. Rockville, MD: American Health Assistance Foundation.

Bahr, M. (1992). *The memory box*. Morton Grove, IL: A. Whitman.

Bauer, M. D. (1999). *An early winter*. Boston: Houghton Mifflin.

Blue, R. (1972). *Grandma didn't wave back*. New York: Watts.

Cargill, K. (1997). *Nana's new home: A comforting story explaining Alzheimer's*. Krisper Publications.

Fox, M. (1985). *Wilfrid Gordon McDonald Partridge*. Brooklyn, NY: Kane/Miller.

Guthrie, D. (1986). *Grandpa doesn't know it's me*. New York: Human Sciences Press.

Holl, K. (1988). *No strings attached*. New York: Atheneum.

Karkowsky, N. (1989). *Grandma's soup*. Rockville, MD: Dar-Ben Copies.

Kelly, B. (1996). *Harpo's horrible secret*. Prairie Grove, AR: Ozark.

Kibbey, M. (1991). *The helping place*. Minneapolis, MN: Carolrhoda Books.

Kibbey, M. (1991). *My Grammy: A book about Alzheimer's disease*. Minneapolis, MN: Lerner Publishing.

Klein, N. (1986). *Going backwards*. New York: Scholastic.

Kroll, V. (1995). *Fireflies, peach pies, and lullabies*. New York: Simon & Schuster.

McIntyre, C. (2005). *Flowers for grandpa Dan: A gentle story to help children understand Alzheimer's disease*. St. Louis, MO: Thumbprint Press.

Nelson, V. M. (1988). *Always gramma*. New York: Scribner.

Potaracke, R. (1994). *Nanny's special gift*. Mahwah, NJ: Paulist Press.

Sanford, D. (1989). *Maria's grandma gets mixed up*. Portland, OR: Multnomah.

Scacco, L. (2005). *Always my Grandpa: A story for children about Alzheimer's disease.* Washington, DC: Magination Press.

Schein, J. (1988). *Forget-me-not.* Toronto: Firefly Books.

Schnurbush, B. (2007). *Striped shirts and flowered pants: A story about Alzheimer's disease for young children.* Washington, DC: Magination Press.

Shawyer, M. (1996). *What's wrong with Grandma?: A family's experience with Alzheimer's.* Amherst, NY: Prometheus Books.

Shriver, M. (2004). *What's happening to Grandpa?* New York: Little, Brown & Co. and Warner Books.

Tolan, S. S. (1978). *Grandpa—and me.* New York: Scribner.

Whitelaw, N. (1991). *A beautiful pearl.* Morton Grove, IL: Albert Whitman.

Wilkinson, B. (1995). *Coping when a grandparent has Alzheimer's disease.* New York: Rosen Publishing.

Willner-Pardo, G. (1999). *Figuring out Frances.* Boston: Houghton Mifflin.

Alzheimer's
Disease Resources

Alzheimer's Association (http://www.alz.org)
24/7 Helpline
Contact for information, referral, and support
800-272-3900
(tdd) 866-403-3073
(e-mail) info@alz.org
National office
225 N. Michigan Ave., Fl. 17
Chicago, IL 60601-7633
312-335-8700
(tdd) 312-335-5886
(fax) 866-699-1246

Alzheimer's Store
3197 Trout Place Road
Cumming, GA 30041
800-752-3238
http://www.alzstore.com

Ableware
Maddak, Inc.
6 Industrial Road
Pequannock, NJ 07440-1993
973-628-7600
http://www.ableware.com

AliMed
297 High Street
Dedham, MA 02026
800-225-2610
http://www.alimed.com

Aspen Publishers, Inc.
200 Orchard Ridge Drive
Gaithersburg, MD 20878
http://www.aspenpub.com

Attainment Company, Inc.
P.O. Box 930160
Verona, WI 53593-0160
800-327-4269
http://www.attainment-inc.com

B. Shackman & Co., Inc. (nostalgia, stickers, cut-outs, books)
85 Fifth Ave. (16th St.)
New York, NY 10003
800-221-7656
http://www.shackman.com

Barry Emons (European materials: Snoezelen, aromatherapy)
Hoefslag 11 5411 LS Zeeland
(tel.) 0486-452626
http://www.barryemons.nl (Dutch only)

Best Alzheimer's Products
877-300-3021
http://www.best-alzheimers-products.com

Briggs Corporation (professional forms)
P.O. Box 1698
Des Moines, IA
50306-1698
800-247-2343
http://www.briggscorp.com

Caregiver's Resource, Inc.
888-791-7301, ext. 81
http://www.caregiverresource.com

Crestwood Company
6625 N. Sidney Place
Milwaukee, WI 53209-3259
414-352-5678
http://www.communicationaids.com

Don Johnston, Inc.
1000 North Rand Road Bldg. 115
P.O. Box 639
Wauconda, IL 60084
800-999-4660
http://www.donjohnston.com

Flaghouse (adults special needs and Snoezelen catalogs)
601 Flaghouse Drive
Hasbrouck Heights, NJ 07604
800-793-7900
http://www.flaghouse.com

Health Professions Press, Inc.
P.O. Box 10624
Baltimore, MD 21285
888-337-8808
http://www.healthpropress.com

Innovative Speech Therapy (therapy, consultations, webinars, seminars, and a free
newsletter)
Potomac, MD 20854
301-602-2899/800-IST-2550
http://www.innovatigvespeech.com

Insight Media (training tapes: *Communicating with Persons with Alzheimer's Disease:
The FOCUSED Program for Caregivers*)
http://www.insight-media.com/

Janelle Publications, Inc. (games)
P.O. Box 811
1189 Twombley Road
Dekalb, IL 60115
800-888-8834
http://www.janellepublications.com/

Lake Solitude Media
232 East 2nd Street, Suite 101
P.O. Box 463
Casper, WY 82602
307-266-4461
http://www.alzheimersbooks.com

LinguiSystems, Inc. (adult rehabilitation and teen books)
3100 4th Avenue East
Moline, IL 61244-9700
800-776-4332 (800-PRO-IDEA)
http://www.linguisystems.com

MedicAlert + Safe Return
(enrollment tel): 1-888-572-8566
(emergency response tel): 1-800-625-3780
http://www.alz.org/care/dementia-medic-alert-safe-return.asp

MindStart.com
Minneapolis, MM
612-868-5831
http://www.mind-start.com

eNASCO (senior activities materials, including life-like dolls)
901 Janesville Ave.
P.O. Box 901
Fort Atkinson, WI 53538
800-558-9595
http://www.enasco.com

National Council of Certified Dementia Practitioners
877-729-5191
http://www.nccdp.org

National Institute on Aging
301-496-1752
http://www.nia.nih.gov

Northern Speech Services, Inc.
325 Meecher Road
Gaylord, MI 49735
888-337-3866
http://www.nss-nrs.com

PRO-ED
8700 Shoal Creek Blvd.
Austin, TX 78757-6897
800-897-3202
http://www.proedinc.com

Video Respite (excellent CDs)
5370 Lake Creek Road
Herber City, Utah 84032
435-657-0255
http://www.videorespite.com

References

Alzheimer's Association. (2012). 2012 Alzheimer's disease facts and figures. *Alzheimer's and Dementia: The Journal of the Alzheimer's Association, 8*, 131–168.

Brackey, J. A. (2007). *Creating moments of joy for the person with Alzheimer's or dementia (4th Ed.)*. West Lafayette: IN: Purdue University Press.

Brown, L. L., & Hammill, D. D. (1990). *Behavior rating profile (2nd Ed.)*. Austin, TX: PRO-ED.

Camp, C. J., Judge, K. S., Bye, C. A., Fox, K. M., Bowden, J., Bell, M., Valencic, K., & Mattern, J. M. (1997). An intergenerational program for persons with dementia using Montessori methods. *The Gerontologist, 37*, 688–692.

Clark, G. M., & Patton, J. R. (1997). *Transition planning inventory*. Austin, TX: PRO-ED.

Conners, C. K. (1997). *Conners' rating acales (Rev. Ed.)*. North Tonawanda, NY: Multi-Health Systems.

Dreher, B. B. (1997). Montessori and Alzheimer's: A partnership that works. *American Journal of Alzheimer's Disease, 12*(3), 138–140.

Eisner, E. (2001). *Can do activities for adults with Alzheimer's disease: Strength-based communication and programming*. Austin, TX: PRO-ED.

Eisner, E. (1999, July 22). What people need to know when visiting relatives in a nursing home. *New Jersey Jewish News*, S-8.

Eisner, E. (1998, May). Mommy, Grandma doesn't know me! *Suburban Parent*, 8–9.

Eisner, E. (1997). Making memories: Tips for families visiting loved ones with Alzheimer's. *ADVANCE for Physician Assistants, 5*(5), 58–60.

Eisner, E. (1996a). Communicating with patients with Alzheimer's disease and dementias. *The Nursing Spectrum, 8A*(25), NJ3.

Eisner, E. (1996b). Enhancing family communication for patients with dementias. *ADVANCE for Speech-Language Pathologists & Audiologists, 6*(20), 8–11.

Eisner, E. (1996c). Helping children to cope with adult's dementia. *ADVANCE for Speech-Language Pathologists & Audiologists, 6*(36), 9.

Gardner, H. (1999). *Intelligence reframed.* New York: Basic Books.

Gardner, H. (1997). *Extraordinary minds: Portraits of exceptional individuals and an examination of our extraordinariness.* NY: Basic Books.

Gardner, H. (1993). *Multiple intelligences: The theory in practice.* NY: Basic Books.

Gardner, H. (1983). *Frames of mind: The theory of multiple intelligences.* NY: Basic Books.

Joltin, A., Camp, D. J, Noble, B. H., & Antenucci, V. M. (2005). *A Different visit: Activities for caregivers and their loved ones with memory impairments.* Beachwood, OH: Myers Research Institute.

Kalb, C. (2000, January 31). Coping with darkness. *Newsweek,* 52–54.

Kindig, M. N., & Carnes, C. (1993). *Coping with Alzheimer's disease and other dementing illness.* San Diego, CA: Singular Publishing Group.

Klosterman, C. (2012, June 24). The ethicist: To tell or not to tell. *New York Times Magazine, 13*

Levine Madori, L. (2007). *Therapeutic thematic arts programming for older adults.* Baltimore, MD: Health Professions Press.

Reisberg, B. (1996). Slowing the progression of Alzheimer's disease (session B7). *Shaping Alzheimer Care: Power of Change* (proceeding book). The Fifth National Alzheimer's Disease Education Conference. Alzheimer's Association. Chicago, Illinois, July 14–17.

Reisberg, B. (1988). Functional assessment staging (FAST). *Psycho-pharmacology Bulletin, 24,* 653–659.

Reisberg, B., Ferris, S. H., de Leon, M. J., & Crook, T. (1982). The global deterioration scale for assessment of primary degenerative dementia. *American Journal of Psychiatry, 139,* 1136–1139.

Ripich, D. N. (2005). *Revised FOCUSED Caregiver's Guide, Communicating with persons with Alzheimer's Disease: The FOCUSED program for Caregivers.* New York: Insight Media.

Terman, L. M. (1916). The measurement of intelligence. Boston: Houghton Mifflin.

Vance, D., Camp, C., Kabacoff, M., & Greenwalt, L. (1996, winter). Montessori methods: Innovative interventions for adults with Alzheimer's disease. *Montessori LIFE,* 10–11.

Index

Note: *f* indicates forms, *g* indicates guides, *t* indicates tables.